Children's Types
Frans Kusse

I dedicate this book to my beloved daughters, Floske and Myrthe,
from whom I learned so much about children, and to Vionne and Roderick,
who from time to time gave me extra lessons.

With many thanks to Gio for love and support and to my father André,
who taught me to always see the good in others,
and to my mother Maria, to whom I owe whatever talent I have for writing.

Children's Types

56 Homeopathic Constitutional Remedies

Frans Kusse

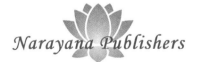

Narayana Publishers

Contents

Children`s Types
56 Homeopathic Constitutional Remedies
Frans Kusse

First English edition 2010

ISBN 978-3-939931-91-1

Title of the Dutch Original:
Wat voor type is mijn kind?
© 2006 Frans Kusse, Amsterdam

Translated by Aidan Constable

Narayana Publishers, Blumenplatz 2, 79400 Kandern, Germany
Tel.: +49 7626 9749700 info@narayana-publishers.eu
www.narayana-publishers.eu

© 2010 Narayana Verlag GmbH

Publisher's Foreword

The old standard work by Borland on homeopathic child types has finally found a worthy modern successor to rework the subject matter and extend it by drawing on the author's own personal experience. People have often asked why there is no book which, apart from describing the well-known major child remedies, also covers the new remedies particularly well-suited to treating children.

We are particularly pleased to be able to offer such a high-quality book to all those interested in homeopathy. Remedies such as *Beryllium, Lithium, Manganum, Helium, Hydrogen,* or *Saccharum* officinale are often indicated for children, but so far they have only been described in the treatment of adults or scattered through the professional journals. The personable Dutch doctor, Dr. Frans Kusse, was ideally suited to such a task due to his extensive clinical experience with children and his tireless commitment. We are now proud to present his successful Dutch work for the first time in English.

Due to the outstanding clinical quality of the book, we did not simply want to leave it at a translation. The high caliber of the 56 remedy descriptions made it worthwhile to enrich the book with photographic portraits — homeopathic typology in particular can benefit from such portraits. From our practice in Kandern, we were able to add 47 photographs of children. Most remedies have two characteristic pictures, which often show astonishing similarities as a pair. These are almost all long-standing cases that responded very well to the remedy in question, mostly repeatedly and with excellent effects when the remedy was given again months or years later.

The first constitutional-typological photographs of homeopathic remedies came from the German doctor, the late Dr. Beuchelt, from whose work several photos are shown here with the kind permission of his family.

We sincerely hope this enchanting book will help all colleagues, interested parents and grandparents, teachers and psychologists to recognize the children's remedies shown!

Kandern, January 2010   *The publisher*

Homeopathy for Children

Self-healing powers

Human beings naturally have the power to heal themselves. This is why most children get better on their own with a bit of attention and some peace and quiet. The immune system of healthy people is able to keep many viruses, bacteria, and other infectious agents at bay. Small wounds normally heal alone. Our body can do a lot on its own!

Suitable for children

There are, however, chronic illnesses that do not simply heal on their own, such as asthma and eczema. There are also children who are unable on their own to overcome certain ailments such as recurring colds, ear infections, bronchitis, and the like. Their bodies clearly do not have the resistance that most children have by nature.

Homeopathy is a type of medicine in which the self-healing power of the body is stimulated. Homeopathic remedies give the body a stimulus to self-healing. This makes it possible to heal many children with recurring illnesses.

This self-healing power is often greater for children than for older people. In a child, everything is young and bursting with energy, including the power of recovery, which is why homeopathy is particularly well suited for children!

Self-treatment with homeopathy

For common and harmless complaints, you can select a homeopathic remedy for your child on your own. Think of coughs, teething complaints, baby colic, diaper rash, colds, and so on. In most countries, you can easily purchase the remedies described in this book.

Homeopathic remedies are produced from natural substances such as plants, minerals, and animal products. Due to the method of preparation — they are diluted and shaken ("succussed"), which we call potentization — the remedies only have an energetic, stimulant action with scarcely any side effects. You can use these remedies with a clear conscience.

About the professional homeopath

You should consult a qualified homeopath for recurring complaints, chronic illnesses and behavioral problems. Homeopathic doctors and many lay homeopaths have a medical as well as a homeopathic training in order to correctly recognize the illness and to competently find the appropriate remedy for your child.

If necessary, conventional medications can be given at the same time as homeopathic remedies. The homeopath may confer with the primary care doctor (the family doctor) or the specialist.

It is less well known that homeopathy can be beneficial for developmental disorders in children. Well-chosen remedies can help stabilize children physically as well as mentally, thereby increasing the chances for growth and development. If children feel comfortable, their demeanor usually also improves.

Introduction to the homeopathic child type

Homeopathy is continually developing and renewing itself. The development in the last twenty years has been at breakneck speed. Thanks to international congresses and modern communication methods, homeopaths worldwide can now exchange ideas far more effectively than in the past.

In 1790, at the time when the German doctor Samuel Hahnemann founded homeopathy, physical illnesses took center stage. Hahnemann had his own methods of observation, and wrote in his book "Organon of the Medical Art" that the psychological symptoms are mostly more important for the choice of remedy than the physical ones. For some remedies, such as *Pulsatilla*, he described the character traits that he often found in people who had been healed by the same remedy.

Many homeopaths have further developed these insights, and assigned types to the most common homeopathic remedies based on character traits. This book describes the most commonly occurring homeopathic child types.

How many types are there?

Every child is ultimately unique — which means there ought to be millions of different remedies, one for each child. Fortunately, it's possible to classify people into types. With the number of remedies described in this book, it's possible to help many children.

Nevertheless, homeopaths are searching for more subtle classifications and actually work with hundreds of specified types. It's impossible to learn every symptom of so many remedies. Homeopaths already discovered in the last century that there are groups of very similar remedies such as, for example, the various plant families. A similar classification is possible for remedies from the mineral kingdom as well as for remedies made from animal products.

Is one remedy enough?

Although there are people who can be cured of deep-seated illnesses by a single remedy, most people in this situation require several remedies.

This is primarily because a homeopathic remedy is rarely one hundred percent suited to a person. As you read this book, you will notice that you partially recognize your child in many different remedy descriptions. For example, it may be that a child with stomach ache is helped by a specific remedy, whereas a different remedy is necessary to clear up long-standing grief and anxiety.

Another reason for this is that there are several "layers." Many people are born with a hereditary predisposition. Therefore, allergies, asthma, and the like usually run in families.

Furthermore, various illnesses and traumatic events can form a new layer. It can be necessary to specifically treat the effects of a childhood illness. An example of this is the youngster with developmental delays ever since he had mumps and who is cured when prescribed *Parotidinum*, a homeopathic remedy (nosode) made from a safe dilution of the mumps virus.

Further disruptive factors can include immunizations, deep-seated emotions such as profound grief or repressed anger, and so on.

For all these causes, there are specific homeopathic remedies available. These have the ability to dissolve blockages that could prevent a full recovery.

No self-treatment

This book is written for all those who are interested in homeopathy and especially for those who want to learn more about the remedy that their child has been given by the homeopath.

While parents are encouraged to treat their children with homeo-pathic remedies for acute (simple, short-term) conditions such as colds, fevers, teething and diarrhea, they should not attempt to treat chronic (long-term) conditions but should instead leave the choice to an expert — a professional homeopath.

The Aconitum napellus Child

Monkshood, Wolf's Bane, Monk's Blood

Plant remedy (Ranunculaceae family)

"Strong, intense, and sensitive"

Origin

This splendid plant with its lovely violet-blue flowers in the shape of a monk's hood can be found in damp places in the mountains.

With people who need *Aconitum*, all symptoms start quickly, are intense and have to do with anxiety and fear. *Aconitum* is usually prescribed for children after a severe shock or an event involving fear of death. An *Aconitum* symptom picture can emerge, for example, if a child had a traumatic birth or experienced a catastrophe or an accident in which the shock still sits deep. *Aconitum* can also work wonders for childhood illnesses involving high fever and anxiety.

Strong and sympathetic

Aconitum children have very independent personalities. They have definite opinions of their own, and they know what they want. They are not, however, as obstinate as *Nux vomica* children, their sense of justice is not so developed as *Causticum* children, and they are not as strongly sympathetic as *Phosphorus* children, although in many ways they resemble these remedy types. "Jack-of-all-trades" often applies to them. They are critical and challenging, yet at the same time open and sympathetic.

Aconitum children believe that people should treat each other well. They show a particular kind of idealism that we often see in remedies of the Ranunculaceae plant family. In their ideal world, people don't abandon one another, and death doesn't exist.

The notion that people can die — let alone that they themselves could die — is unbearable for them. If they experience something related to death, they get into a panic. The very same energy that normally helps them get their own way is then expressed as anxiety. The concern that they feel for others and the oversensitivity to bad news are also related to this issue.

12

They want to keep things under control, and therefore also feel responsible for the people around them.

Sensitive nervous system

Although they appear strong and independent on the outside, *Aconitum* children also have an inner sensitivity. But they don't let on about this. They perceive all sensory stimuli such as light and noises intensely. Above all, when they don't feel well, they can't tolerate any noise at all. *Aconitum* children are deeply moved by music that they love.

Their (over-)sensitivity makes it difficult for them to be touched, especially when they're ill. When in pain, they can panic wildly and scream the house down. This reaction is related to the loss of control over their own body. Their body behaves in a way that they don't understand and don't want, which is why they lose their natural confidence. They are panic-stricken and react with complete despair to their powerlessness. Their behavior might even revert to an earlier stage so that, for example, they want to be carried, although they don't want to be comforted. *Aconitum* children can then become very nasty and express their emotions in the form of temper tantrums. What's more, everything that hasn't been dealt with during the day can break out in full force as dreadful images and nightmares at night.

Shock and fear of death

What mostly upsets *Aconitum* children are situations of fear. The fear can be triggered by an awful event such as a serious accident or a fire, but also by a sudden illness, high fever, an operation, or a difficult birth. Even bad news can precipitate an *"Aconitum* state" in susceptible children.

The fear can be so intense and violent that they often think they will soon die. Sometimes they then actually say: "Mum, I'm going to die." They're convinced of it! For small children who can't yet speak, the anxiety can be expressed in various physical symptoms such as urine retention. Older children can express the anxiety as bed-wetting. Fortunately, *Aconitum* is able to remove the fear and resulting complaints and to restore the previous balance.

13

Without suitable treatment, an acute state of anxiety can become chronic, resulting in, for example, fear of crowds, claustrophobia, fear of crossing the street, fear of suffocation, or fear of the future. We often see these fears in children who suffer from hyperventilation. The causes can be varied, but they are almost always concerned with fear of death. *Aconitum* is, therefore, one of the most important remedies for panic attacks with hyperventilation.

Case report

A colleague told me of an *Aconitum* case that graphically demonstrates its use. At a homeopathy course, he had learned that it was a good idea to always carry a vial of *Aconitum* in your pocket. Since then, he had taken this advice to heart. One day, a mother stormed into his practice with her bloodstained son. He had a gash on his hand and was completely beside himself. The cut had to be stitched — but how can you do that with a panic-stricken child? The doctor reached into his pocket and took out the vial of *Aconitum*. He gave the child a few globules and began to prepare his instruments. When he turned round again, he was amazed to see the youngster had calmed down and was talking with his mother. The local anesthetic and even the stitching of the wound were no longer a problem.

Physical symptoms

The physical complaints are also intensely acute and start violently. *Aconitum* is a typical remedy for illnesses that begin very suddenly. Retention of urine (urination is impossible or incomplete) in a newborn is a symptom that can indicate *Aconitum*. This together with the symptoms of delivery (shock, panic, and chill) leads to the *Aconitum* picture.

Aconitum covers complaints due to chill, especially in a cold, dry wind when the weather is otherwise warm. Sudden weakness or fever with severe anxiety is possible after suppressed sweat (for example, due to a chill or the use of an antiperspirant). It is one of the most important remedies for flu, and is the first remedy for inflammation with fever. *Aconitum* is strongly indicated if the ill child does not want to be touched. It can also be very useful for pseudocroup, especially when the child reacts to the constriction with panic.

The pains can be intense, reducing the child to despair. Especially the pain in the nerves can cause them to shriek. Bright red bleeding and burning or numbness and prickling can occur. Sensory perceptions can be felt more intensely and can disturb the child.

Food and Drink

Aconitum children often love cold water, sour food, and bitter drinks. They usually do not tolerate milk well.

The Agaricus muscarius Child

Fly Agaric, Bug Agaric, Fly Amanita

Plant remedy (Agaricaceae family)

"Unrestrained children"

Origin

Agaricus muscarius (or *Amanita muscaria*) is the Latin name for the red fly agaric, the well-known red cap fungus with white spots. It looks harmless, but is far from it. It's known that the Vikings ingested it before they went on their raids of pillage and plunder. Under the influence of the fly agaric, the calm and introverted Scandinavians were transformed into bloodthirsty tyrants who terrorized large areas of Europe. The same fungus was used in olden times for various rituals and an extract is currently one of the so-called "smart drugs."

When studying this remedy, Hahnemann used among other things the precise descriptions of a doctor from Napoleon's army. The army doctor accompanied a group of soldiers who ended up starving in a wood after the slaughter at the Berezina. Having nothing else to eat, the soldiers seized on the fly agaric. They behaved as if they were drunk. Several began to sing and babble, others ran agitatedly around, raising their legs much higher than necessary. Small hurdles appeared to them as huge barriers, and everything seemed to be much bigger than it really was.

Energy

Agaricus children have an incredible amount of energy. So long as this energy is directed and balanced, they are active children who enjoy life. They are happy and open by nature. They wear their heart on their sleeve and like to sing when happy. Their spontaneity expresses itself in practical jokes that they like to play on people, although they aren't primarily seeking attention or recognition. They simply like having fun and love the entertainment. They don't like sitting still and keeping quiet for long periods unless really necessary.

16

Sometimes they don't know when to stop, since they lack boundaries. Then they exaggerate their pranks so much that no one finds them funny anymore. They're extremely talkative and hardly let anyone else get a word in. Listening is often extremely difficult for them; they do not reply to every question they are asked.

The energy that they can generate when angry is enormous. In a rage, their physical strength increases so much that they're capable of feats of strength that would not normally be expected from a child. The extraordinary performance of people in life-threatening situations is well-known — *Agaricus* children are even capable of such exceptional physical feats in less threatening situations.

Sensitive to criticism and punishment

It's important for *Agaricus* children to be taken seriously and to be accepted for what they are. They're particularly sensitive to criticism. They easily feel rebuffed and can react very intensely to criticism and reprimand. If a child becomes ill after being reprimanded or suddenly starts making errors in reading or writing, the homeopathic doctor will quickly think of *Agaricus*.

When these children become disturbed due to physical illness or emotional difficulty, they become hard to stop. They can't focus their energy, and their agitation makes it difficult to concentrate and to learn. They're constantly on the move and sitting still is very difficult for them. They no longer have their movements completely under control, and even muscle jerks can occur due to over-stimulation of the nervous system. Then they often retreat into their own world to the point of completely shutting off from the outside world. If a child is late learning to walk and talk, this can be an extra hint for *Agaricus*.

Invincible warriors or spineless victims

So long as their physical and emotional powers are directed purposefully, they can move mountains and also help other children in difficult situations. But when they become unsettled, their energies — apart from being uninhibited — often lack purpose, although at such times they certainly don't give an impression of strength. They feel weak and frustrated, are emotionally exhausted, and increasingly unable to find solutions. Their speech becomes less controlled and more unclear, and their movements show loss of control. They run the danger of no longer being taken seriously, which just makes things worse as they're still really sensitive to criticism! Instead of the invincible warrior, their true nature, they now come across as spineless victims. Homeopathically prepared *Agaricus* reawakens the old powers.

Reckless and playful

The recklessness of *Agaricus* children is striking. There are few things that they're afraid of. In their lack of inhibition, they're blind to danger and can pull off the most foolhardy stunts. One problem that I've frequently noticed is that, in their over-enthusiasm and restlessness, they know no boundaries. They can't stop talking and messing around. This upsets other children and then what happens is precisely what they wanted to avoid: they're no longer taken seriously and are even ridiculed by the other children.

Death

Children who need *Agaricus* are attracted by dying people. Everything about death engages them. They're afraid of death, but simultaneously fascinated by it. If they themselves are missing something, they want to talk about it with someone else. If something that moves them is being discussed, they can drive others mad with their anxious questions. Then they want to be supported and comforted. In this state, they cry easily and copiously.

Physical symptoms

Agaricus children freeze easily and tolerate cold poorly. If a storm is approaching, their complaints worsen. The morning is their worst time. They feel better in the evening and are in their element when peacefully pursuing some activity.

Agaricus is an important remedy for various neurological illnesses, especially when accompanied by jerking and cramps in the muscles. Facial tics lead the homeopathic doctor to consider this remedy first of all. A typical symptom of *Agaricus* is also that pressure on the vertebrae can trigger involuntary fits of laughter.

Symptoms that fit *Agaricus* are stumbling, walking with too long a stride, clumsy movements, things slipping from the hands, and so on. It's as if the movements are uninhibited and out of control. Diagonal complaints are also a typical symptom of *Agaricus*, such as pains in the left arm and at the same time in the right leg.
They like warmth and sun, although this often gives them headaches. The mucous membranes in their nose can often be very dry, and it's striking that coughing often ends in sneezing.
Agaricus is one of the most important remedies for frostbite of the hands and feet.

Food and Drink

Agaricus children often have a changeable relationship to food. They're either constantly hungry or they have a poor appetite. They tolerate cold drinks and food poorly, although they may ask for them. Bread and eggs are foods that they either love or loathe.

The Alumina Child

Pure clay (Aluminum oxide, Al_2O_3)

Mineral remedy

"Need to form their own identity"

Origin

The metal aluminum is one of the most commonly occurring metals on the earth. Approximately 7.5% of the earth's crust consists of aluminum. The remedy *Alumina* is the aluminum compound (aluminum oxide) that is so far the most commonly used in homeopathy, although pure aluminum is now also being used as a remedy called *Aluminum metallicum*. Clay consists mainly of aluminum oxide, so the characteristics of clay are helpful for us to sketch the remedy.

Mainly a developmental phase

There are some striking symptoms that make us think of *Alumina* for a child. *Alumina* corresponds to a particular developmental phase of the child, rather than to a particular type. Constipation, dry skin, and dullness are the most common symptoms for *Alumina* babies and small children. An additional hint is strong itching, in which they scratch till they bleed, although there's no visible skin eruption. With older children, it's clear that they adapt strongly to their environment and it's difficult for them to develop their own will. Therefore, they're easy to get along with, but they have little "identity of their own." If children find it difficult to become individuals due to fear of being rejected by the group, *Alumina* can strengthen their willpower. Then they'll be able to find their own place in the group and stick to it.

Forming their own identity

Alumina does not so much indicate the type of the child as the developmental phase that it's passing through. *Alumina* refers to the development of a separate identity. This phase belongs to early life. A certain "self-awareness" has developed (this doesn't exist or hardly at all for small children), but it's not yet clear how the child will relate to other people. If during this period the necessary stimulus is missing, the child gets "stuck." It does not develop a clear identity of its own. The picture that the child has of itself remains blurred.

The *Alumina* phase is to do with setting the boundaries of the bodies that we inhabit in relation to those of other people.

Fitting in to the environment

Since *Alumina* children are thoroughly convinced that they belong somewhere, but neither know what role to take nor how to do so, they just fit in. This makes them too docile as children. They can take on any shape and are as "malleable as unfired clay." They're convinced that it's good to fit in with others and regard it as egotistical to simply get their own way. Their adaptation consists of just adopting the thoughts and habits of others. Behind this is the fear of being abandoned if they demand too much space for themselves, but also the idea that it's not good to pursue your own ideas.

So long as they have relationships with well-meaning children and adults, everything is fine. The danger is that they're not clear what they want for themselves, so that others will repeatedly fill this gap for them.

In search of themselves

Since their own will is not very strongly developed, these children are very easily influenced. *Alumina* children quickly have the feeling of doing something wrong. They can't imagine that other children do not mean well toward them. When they notice that the intentions of others towards them are sometimes less than pure, this annoys them, but it's doubtful whether they'll show their anger.

This state of affairs can encourage them to stand up for themselves more, and to start the search for who they really are and what they want!

Only one task at a time

Alumina children can be slow to think and act. It's as if they get stuck. Since they're aware of their sluggishness, an inner feeling of harassment can develop. It's very difficult for them to do two things

21

at once, such as to do something with the hands while talking at the same time. They need all their attention to perform a single task. Everything should occur at their pace and in their own way. *Alumina* children get into a panic when too much is demanded of them.

Identification with the other person

When *Alumina* children become unsettled, this can upset them. They've identified so closely with the other person that they're no longer able to distinguish what they themselves want, and what the other person wants. They end up doubting themselves and asking themselves: "Did I say that or did my friend?" If the confusion increases, *Alumina* children can get the feeling that they are merging with the other person and that there are no more boundaries between themselves and other people. Everything seems unreal.

Fear of their own impulses

Since it's so difficult for them to establish contact with themselves, they're often afraid of what's inside them. Can they trust themselves? Fear of knives is characteristic of *Alumina*. For no reason, they're afraid that they could harm themselves. They're afraid of going mad. *Alumina* can help these children to get in touch with themselves and to become grounded.

Physical symptoms

Alumina children are mostly warm-blooded, and tolerate heat and dryness poorly. On the other hand, moisture is good for them. If you take them with you into the mountains, you'll notice that their complaints get worse. Their worst time is 09:00 (9 a.m.).

Despite the aggravation from warmth, they don't like winter either. They easily get a cold and take a long time to recover since their resistance is poor. Sluggishness, weakness, paralysis, and dryness are four symptoms that accompany all complaints.

Sluggishness occurs in the esophagus — they have difficulty swallowing their food. There's also sluggishness in the bladder — urination takes a long time — and in the gut. We see constipation more commonly in *Alumina* babies than in older *Alumina* children.

Everything is dry: the eyes, the mouth, the throat, the gut. The skin can also be extremely dry with much itching, although there's no visible external irritation.

Food and Drink

Alumina children have a special relationship to potatoes: they either really want them or they have a strong dislike of them. Eating potatoes worsens their complaints. They love dry food, rice, and pastries. *Alumina* children can crave indigestible things such as charcoal, clay and the like — as if they want to make up for what they're missing.

They hate meat and tolerate processed foods poorly. A natural diet is best for everyone, but for *Alumina* children it's an absolute must.

The Ammonium carbonicum Child

Ammonium carbonate, Hartshorn salt, $(NH_4)_2CO_3$

Mineral remedy

"Strong identification with the father figure"

Origin

Hahnemann was not only a doctor, but also a great chemist. In his book "The Chronic Diseases," he describes precisely how he derived the salt ammonium carbonate from ammonia and sodium carbonate. He healed many patients with this. Until ten years ago, we knew *Ammonium carbonicum* only as a remedy for old people with asthmatic complaints or chronic bronchitis. We didn't know which type corresponds to this remedy, let alone which child type. It has since become one of the most commonly prescribed remedies, especially for pubescent children.

Idealization of the father

At a young age, *Ammonium carbonicum* children tend to idealize everything about their father. Their father is the biggest, strongest, most intelligent, and best father in the whole world. He can do everything and he knows everything. The "father" need not be the biological father — he can also be someone who takes on the role of father, such as the stepfather or the schoolteacher. So long as they have a good relationship with their father, they can cope with anything. Their nature shows through clearly when they're disappointed by someone they are close to. But they're most deeply affected when their idealized image of the father breaks down.

Grudge

The *Ammonium carbonicum* picture doesn't only show anger. It goes deeper — grudge, resentment, and sometimes even hate are what come to mind when these children can describe their emotions. We mostly get the description from one of the parents. The way they sit in the doctor's room speaks volumes. *Ammonium carbonicum* children are reluctant to speak when they're injured or furious. They stare rigidly ahead, and are completely disinclined to contribute anything whatsoever to the subject of discussion. They themselves don't experience this as a problem, but those around them certainly do. They loll around on their chair, scarcely answering a single question. When they come to the doctor, it's due to a chronic cold, a sinus infection, or skin problems — on no account because they don't feel well in themselves. What a ludicrous idea!

Disappointed

The more strongly a person is idealized, the bigger the disappointment when it turns out they are neither strong nor all-knowing. Therefore, *Ammonium carbonicum* children are hurt more deeply than most other children when they discover that their father is just an ordinary person. Other children can get into an *Ammonium carbonicum* state when the behavior of the father figure deviates strongly from their expectations. We see this picture, for example, in children who have been emotionally or physically abused by their father. But for children with a predisposition to the *Ammonium carbonicum* type, a "straightforward" disappointment is enough to evoke this picture. The ideal breaks down and they convert the disappointment and pain into resentment and hate, rather than feel the underlying sorrow. They express these feelings through stubborn silence, and they become sarcastic, ranting and swearing freely. Yet the rage is locked inside and can turn into a silent and gloomy disposition. They are then difficult to reach, remaining in their own fantasy world, and concentration is difficult for them.

Fighting for an ideal or against injustice

Society with all its prescriptions and authorities corresponds metaphorically to the father figure. Everything that happens there is observed and judged in the same way as with the father. If they're unfairly treated at school or in part-time work, the result is similar, since the teaching staff or employers also represent a kind of father figure. In puberty, many *Ammonium carbonicum* children take up the fight against injustice, corruption, and abuse of power in the world. They're typical "angry young men" — rebels and radicals. Others

25

might work in an environmental group or help people in need, asylum seekers, and so on.

Don't get me wrong: their dedication to these aims is important and valuable but it can't free them from their inner suffering. This will express itself in many roundabout ways, either by emotional signals or physical symptoms. The protest against the established order is also noticeable as lack of interest, provocative clothing, or sloppy appearance. In this they're similar to *Sulfur* children. Whereas for *Sulfur* this comes from laziness and for the sake of convenience, it's to do with protest for *Ammonium carbonicum* children.

Physical symptoms

Most complaints occur on the right side of the body. *Ammonium carbonicum* children are generally chilly — many complaints arise from the cold or are worsened by it. A noticeable symptom is a temporary loss of memory following a bang or blow to the head.

Colds, which they catch easily, can be accompanied by a corrosive nasal discharge that turns into maxillary sinusitis (on the right). This can also affect the lungs, especially in the elderly.

Food and Drink

Ammonium carbonicum children feel better after eating. They love candy, especially chocolate, but also sour things. We often find a dislike of meat. They mostly cannot tolerate potatoes.

The Anacardium Child

Marking nut, Malacca nut, Cashew nut

Plant remedy (Anacardiaceae family)

"An angel and a devil"

Origin

There are two types of *Anacardium,* a western one (occidental) native to South America and an eastern one (oriental) native to India. *Anacardium occidentale* is made from the seed of the cashew tree, the well-known cashew nut. This is a kidney-shaped nut that was used in the past to rejuvenate and refresh the facial skin. Experience has shown that it's best to wash the hands after handling the nut, since otherwise a strong, itchy skin rash can develop.

Anacardium orientale is used more often in homeopathy, and is therefore the one described here. The nut is heart-shaped, which explains why the Latin name *Anacardium* is used, as this means "like a heart." The two nuts have such similar pictures that it's difficult to distinguish them. For skin complaints, *Anacardium occidentale* (Cashew) probably works better. The fact that *Anacardium* has two variants from two different places on the earth is characteristic for the remedy — this dichotomy is a central theme running through the remedy picture.

Two sides

Anacardium children combine two opposite characteristics. For example, they can be well-behaved, model schoolchildren who work hard and do everything asked of them. In familiar surroundings, however, the other side of their character comes to light. At home, they can let out their anger on their brother or sister, be cheeky to their parents, or play unexpected, sneaky tricks. The little angel known to the outside world can turn into a little devil at home.

Obviously, every child combines different characteristics and the outside world always sees a different aspect from the people who live together with the child. But for *Anacardium* children the gap is

27

particularly wide — as if the light and dark sides have no connection with each other.

Need to prove themselves

The natural self-confidence of *Anacardium* children can be destroyed by external influences. Due to the resulting extreme inner doubt, *Anacardium* children live under constant pressure to succeed. They want to always show that they can fulfill the expectations of them, and want to prove themselves by their performance. Behind this there is a deep uncertainty and doubt about their self-worth. When they're old enough to talk about it, many will perhaps say that they don't think they have much self-worth or even that they're worthless. But most children have difficulty putting this into words. They've developed a thick skin, hoping in this way to avoid being hurt.

When things get serious, such as before an exam, they become unbelievably tense. *Anacardium* was always, even before we discovered its full homeopathic picture, one of the most important remedies for exam nerves. The doubt can express itself as a difficulty in making up one's mind. They either postpone decisions or they decide categorically and immediately so as to banish all doubt.

Anacardium children tend to be clearer about what they don't want than they are about what they do want.

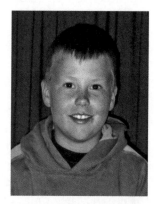

Anac.

Separation

There is mostly a clear cause for the personality of *Anacardium* children. At some time in their lives, usually in the early years, there was a separation. The separation can have occurred either in the outside world, in their inner world, or both. Perhaps the parents often had violent rows or there was a separation or a divorce.

If the personalities of the mother and father are quite different, this can lead to an inner conflict in the children. They want to keep the parents together, which is, however, an impossible task. The "solution" is to split oneself. Their disappointment and their fury emerge not at all, incompletely, or only in unobserved moments. They prefer peace and quiet. Therefore, *Anacardium* children can become over-zealous supporters of the peace movement, or they can join a non-violent group when they're older. So long as their fury and frustration are not conscious, these remain hidden and can break out unexpectedly.

High demands

Another cause for the emergence of the *Anacardium* picture is the excessive expectations that one or both parents have of their child. The children try to fulfill these expectations, but get caught in a conflict when they do not receive the recognition they're seeking. This conflict can be expressed in a variety of ways. They either become very quiet and withdrawn, full of self-doubt, or they get stuck into their work so that the outside world doesn't notice how unsure they really are. They badly want to prove themselves.

In the long run, this attitude causes physical complaints. The inner conflict can lead to a slowing down of their development compared to other children. Their powers of concentration and memory can decline. The emotional tension of having to perform eventually becomes too much for them. As already mentioned, tests and exams are the point at which all their tensions are externalized, and there is a great danger that *Anacardium* children then come to grief.

The dark side

When *Anacardium* children lose heart, they can show unimaginable fury and become indifferent to others. To start with, they sometimes play the clown, although they can't tolerate being laughed at or told off. Their behavior can be very changeable.

Later on, their conduct can become spiteful, challenging, and aggressive. They rant, swear, and can even be really mean to other children or grown-ups. It's as if they're trying to alleviate their own pain by causing suffering in others. Initially they still regret their behavior, but later they don't even seem to have feelings of guilt. Deliberately destroying things, hurting other children — it can go

29

much too far. We can only understand their behavior when we immerse ourselves in their world in order to appreciate how they experience events in their life.

Physical symptoms

Many physical complaints worth mentioning for *Anacardium* are the result of frustration and unassimilated emotions, such as fury that they can't express, anxiety (with tests and exams!), and nervousness. Repressed skin rashes (for example, due to allopathic medications) can be a further cause of physical symptoms.

There are some physical symptoms that *Anacardium* as well as *Lycopodium* children show. The time of day when *Anacardium* children feel worst is the same, namely from 16:00 to 20:00 (4 to 8 p.m.). The pains also often begin for both on the right side and then spread over to the left. Since there are very many points of similarity ("at school an angel, at home a rascal"), these two remedies are easily mixed up.

Due to tension and nervousness, *Anacardium* children can often end up with a diminished sense of smell, hearing, or sight. It seems as if their nerves fail. The inner tension can also lead to external trembling so that they get really shaky knees. The trembling can also be caused by physical exertion. They are so weak from exhaustion that they can scarcely stay on their feet or walk up the stairs. Joints and tendons are sensitive parts of the body, as is the nervous system in general.

Anacardium children suffer from a feeling of emptiness in the stomach, independent of the time of day. This feeling is temporarily improved — as are many other symptoms — by eating.

Anacardium children can suffer from various skin complaints, from eczema to warts, blisters, and growths. The mostly very intense itching is worsened by scratching and relieved by hot water. *Anacardium* belongs to the same plant family as poison ivy (the source of the remedy *Rhus tox)*; both remedies are useful for poison ivy. In general, *Anacardium* children are sensitive to dampness and cold, and feel better with warmth. Many complaints are worsened by movement.

The Antimonium crudum Child

Stibnite, Antimony sulfide Sb₂S₃

Mineral remedy

"Contrary"

Origin

Antimonium crudum is a mineral that has long been used in homeopathy. It is a compound of the metal antimony (stibium – Sb) and sulfur (sulfide). The pure form of antimony, *Antimonium metallicum*, has only recently been used in homeopathy.

In terms of its effects and its external form, the metal has many similarities with arsenic. It's a silver-white, highly shiny, brittle, metallic substance that is easily pulverized, and mostly occurs as a compound of sulfur (sulfide) or oxygen (oxide). Nowadays, we use antimony sulfide in lead-antimony batteries, zinc alloys, pyrotechnics, and for the manufacture of textiles, rubber, and glass.

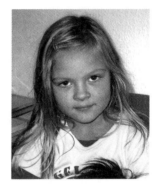

Ant-c.

Antimonium crudum is extracted from a natural mineral, needle antimony (stibnite). In the Ichinokawa mine on the Japanese island of Shikoku, stibnite is found in the form of crystals up to 2 feet (60 cm) high and 2 inches (5 cm) wide. Due to their shape, they are often used in Japan as fence posts. The crystals characteristically form at right angles to the earth's magnetic field.

The name "antimony" comes from the Greek *"antimonos,"* which means "against loneliness." Antimony was discovered in 1450, when chemists were still alchemists.

Irritable babies

Antimonium crudum has various different aspects. Children who need this remedy are sentimental and vulnerable. But as long as they still can't speak, they express their discontent very intensely. They can react furiously to any kind of attention and contact, and they do not want to be washed. Their digestive tract is very sensitive and works very slowly, so that they often belch and even vomit breast milk. When they are being weaned, they often won't tolerate any-one else in the room. They suffer from contagious impetigo, skin rashes on the head, and chronic inflammation of the eye. For new-borns with these symptoms together with ill-temper and irritabil-ity, *Antimonium crudum* is well-indicated. *Antimonium crudum* regulates their digestion and their mood also improves, since they're basically yearning for love and attention.

Dreamers

When *Antimonium crudum* children are feeling well, they can have fabulous daydreams and are very romantic. Their favorite clothes are tasteful and correspond to their sensitive character. Their dreams are not unrealistic, but are often hard to realize in this dif-ficult world. When they get a little older — although even very young children can feel these emotions strongly — they like fantasizing about being in love. Moonlight reinforces their sentimental feelings.

A gift for music

Most *Antimonium crudum* children are musically gifted or at least receptive to music. When they can freely choose a music instru-ment, they frequently opt for the flute. The "crosswise" or "con-trary" aspect of this instrument is something we find reflected in all other areas.

It's important for these children to be able to develop their musical or other creative talents. The longing to demonstrate their artistic side to the public is very strong — also because in this way they can win the attention and love that they yearn for.

In everything that they do, it's important to them to do it properly. In their creativity, they demand the best of themselves and are not easy to please. Deep inside, they fear that they can't perform as necessary to fulfill the role expected of them.

Self-Critical

This anxiety makes them sensitive to the least criticism. They have the feeling that others are getting in their way and are offended by the slightest thing. Since they're very self-critical, a trifle can be enough to make them feel rejected. For this reason, they're extremely sensitive to the behavior of their parents and teachers. Disapproval feeds their inner doubt and arouses resistance, whereas encouragement strengthens their self-image.

Antimonium crudum children have a strong will, and can become "eccentrics" if they're unable to act according to their own judgment.

Stubborn and contrary

When they feel offended by negative criticism or rejection, they throw in the towel. Nothing satisfies them and any attention, every look or touch, can arouse rage. Their anger is directed to the outside world, and then no one can do anything right. *Antimonium crudum* helps these gifted people to love themselves once more!

The tendency to challenge is a leitmotiv of their lives, just as the stibnite crystal arranges itself crosswise — or in a contrary way — to the earth's magnetic field. "Contrary" also means being different from other people or being a one-off (one of a kind). It's characteristic that they choose something as unique as the flute. So long as they're in balance, this "being unique" is a character trait that distinguishes them; as a reaction to inner frustration, however, it can lead to isolation.

Loneliness

It's impossible to say with certainty whether the oversensitivity of an *Antimonium crudum* child is innate or is due to trauma. The behavior of *Antimonium crudum* children can easily lead to loneliness, from which they find it hard to emerge without help. Behind their moody, irritable and rude exterior, there is often a hidden sadness, which they express more easily after a dose of *Antimonium crudum*. While researching the remedy for this book, it became quite clear to me why the alchemists called this metal "against aloneness."

Physical symptoms

Antimonium crudum children are often quite stout, coarse, and tend toward being overweight. Complaints occur frequently on the left side.

They tend not to tolerate warmth so well since they are by nature mostly warm. They react poorly to radiant heat in particular. The warmth from an oven can give them a headache or cause coughing. They prefer fresh air and they sweat at the least exertion.

On the other hand, they can get all sorts of complaints from being chilled by cold water, such as headaches, vomiting, or diarrhea.

When *Antimonium crudum* children don't feel well, they tend to eat far too much, which can cause stomach and gut symptoms. One typical symptom of this remedy is a tongue with a thick white coating.

Further complaints that can occur are an excessive production of saliva, bleeding gums, and mouth ulcers. A unique symptom, very typical for *Antimonium crudum*, is the simultaneous occurrence of pains in the stomach and in the legs.

Antimonium crudum has a strong effect on the skin and is known for its curative effects in hardening and hornification (thickening) such as (painful) calluses on the soles of the feet, corns, and warts. Cracks at various places, such as the nostrils, frequently occur. It's as if the skin were building a shield against the outer world.

Food and Drink

Antimonium crudum children often have a pronounced preference for certain foods, yet paradoxically react to them with oversensitivity. They have a strong desire for sour food, especially for cucumber and pickled gherkins. They also like fruit, raw food, alcohol, sweet things, fat, spices, and cold drinks. They often have an aversion to eggs and bread.

The Apis mellifica Child

Honey bee. Animal remedy

"Busy bee"

Origin

The honey bee, which is used to produce the homeopathic remedy *Apis mellifica*, is an extraordinary insect. Of all the insects on earth, it's the only one that forms a relationship to humans. It also provides honey, a valuable foodstuff. Honey metaphorically represents the wealth of a country (just like milk, which most *Apis* children are crazy about), as in the phrase "a land of milk and honey." Bees have abilities that we only otherwise find in higher mammals. They have an excellent capacity for learning and deduction. The organization and activity in a beehive demonstrate the disciplined character of this little animal. All beekeepers know that beneath the woolly softness and good-natured character of the bee, there's a noticeable sting. But when they're handled with the necessary respect and receive recognition for their work, the honey bee swears enduring allegiance to the beekeeper.

Performance and recognition

The picture of the industrious bee corresponds in a figurative sense to the children for whom this remedy fits. *Apis* children are friendly and helpful. It's part of their nature to give their best, and they work diligently in order to gain some recognition. Of course, this behavior can be reinforced by their parents with their own expectations, but it can often come from the children themselves. They refuse to laze around, and when they do something, they have to do it well. *Apis* children do not need to be pushed to perform. They sense when something is expected of them and get straight down to work. They can work hard, but their way of working may be rather chaotic. These children should be encouraged to take a break and not have such high expectations of themselves.

Sensitive to touch

Although *Apis* children show their reactions in a direct way, they are nevertheless quite reserved and don't like direct contact. Before they embark on a relationship, they must have a sense of reliability and trust. The sensitivity of the skin to touch also has a symbolic meaning. In general, they're not cuddly children like *Pulsatilla* or *Phosphorus* children. Yet their reserve isn't as strong as, for example, *Natrium muriaticum* children, who fear emotional injury. *Apis* children tend to be courageous rather than to disclose their emotions. They've learned to behave strongly and independently, and they rarely show their distress in tears. Anger mostly appears when they're alone — and then a plate or a glass can get smashed. On the other hand, *Apis* children tolerate physical pain poorly and find it hard to cover it up. Although they don't normally get furious or aggressive, they can certainly react very strongly when necessary.

Exam nerves

When they have to prove themselves and achieve good results, they come under pressure. For years, they can dream of failing an exam that they have in fact long ago passed. Moreover, they also have a special solution for situations in which they doubt themselves: they behave as if it doesn't interest them at all!

Apis children cling to their possessions and, therefore, fear losing something. This might be a toy or friends. Their jealousy is connected to this fear. Bees leave their "houses" only when absolutely necessary and are by nature reliable. They don't like change and have a somewhat conservative character.

I'm not ill

Apis children cannot tolerate being ill. They deny their symptoms as long as possible, although they're strongly affected because they're so sensitive. In this respect, they're like *Arnica* children. They tolerate pain very poorly, and when they're in pain, it seems to be much more intense than for others. Maybe this is why they're afraid of pointed objects — due to fear of being pricked.

They rarely express emotions, preferring instead to repress them. This can go so far that they appear to be numb. They become apathetic and hardly show reactions any more. With *Apis* and the right kind of support, they can learn once more to admit their emotions and become the lively children that they basically are.

Physical symptoms

The best-known physical symptoms for *Apis* bring to mind a bee sting: swelling and burning pains. The feeling of swelling can occur all over the body: on the skin, in the mouth, in the neck, or in the tummy. In children, these swellings are mostly caused by inflammations, such as a throat infection or an allergic reaction.

Warmth and touch worsen the complaints, whereas cold improves them.

Food and Drink

It's noticeable that *Apis* children react sensitively to the color of food, just as bees prefer particular colors in flowers. A special characteristic with fever is that they're still not thirsty. They have a desire for sour things and milk. They feel better after drinking milk.

The Argentum nitricum Child

Lunar caustic, Silver nitrate ($AgNO_3$)

Mineral remedy

"I want to show that I'm gifted... if it just wasn't for the stage fright"

Origin

Silver nitrate was until recently given to newborn babies to protect their eyes against certain diseases, and has been used in medicine for a long time. This is why *Argentum nitricum* was proved as a remedy right at the beginning of the homeopathic era.

Although in many respects similar to the picture of *Argentum metallicum* (pure silver), *Argentum nitricum* (silver nitrate) has its own specific symptoms, which make it easy to recognize in children.

Fear of failure

Argentum nitricum children possess enough self-confidence and are able to give a good account of themselves. They have a sensitive nature and are sweet-tempered, which makes them vulnerable. They find it hard to put up with rudeness and unjustified, crushing criticism. They want to play an important role, and do this in a lively way if their self-confidence is well-developed. Their urge to be seen and heard is considerable and encompasses not just knowledge, but also artistic expression such as song, music, and painting. When their self-esteem is wounded, however, they turn into shy and withdrawn children, and become silent. The most varied fears can appear, from fear of heights to fear of cancer and of dying. These are often irrational fears. The most striking is the fear of failure. From fear of making mistakes, they no longer want to express themselves.

Connoisseurs of life

Argentum nitricum children are pleasure-seekers and it shows. They are spontaneous, open, happy, and warm-hearted. In society, they

38

are hard to miss. Their interest for others is well-meaning and they can empathize well with the troubles of other people. But then it's important for them to speak about things in order to come to terms with the suffering of others.

Tasty food and drink are pleasurable things. Going out and being seen is very important for somewhat older *Argentum nitricum* children. For this, they prefer an artistic, cultivated environment. They feel drawn to the soft side of art, to music and painting. Even very young *Argentum nitricum* children can be interested in the big questions of life and can make decisions from a strong sense of conviction, such as to become a vegetarian.

Necessary space

Argentum nitricum children need space to fulfill themselves and to be seen. *Argentum nitricum* people typically like going to concerts, but sit at the edge of the row so that they can get out at any time. In children, this is possibly less apparent, but in the cinema or the theater, they automatically look for places that are spacious and roomy. They generally feel better outside in the open air. In a crowd or in a small room, they feel enclosed. Claustrophobia, the fear of enclosed spaces, always makes us think of *Argentum nitricum*.

A further aspect is that they need space metaphorically. They have great difficulty tolerating external pressure, whether to do with meetings or time in general. Older *Argentum nitricum* children say that they have difficulties with appointments, because their time feels restricted. When a meeting is fixed, it's always on their mind, sometimes for hours in advance. They feel rushed and, since they definitely want to be punctual, they usually arrive far too early for their appointments. *Argentum nitricum* is, therefore, one of the most important remedies for anticipatory anxiety, especially when the point in time is fixed.

Stage fright

Argentum nitricum is, together with *Gelsemium*, the most commonly prescribed remedy for stage fright. The desire to present something and thereby to shine is great, but on the other hand they can't tolerate the associated pressure. The difficulty with performances is that a strict schedule must be followed. Everything is fixed and they can't get away from it.

In addition, *Argentum nitricum* children have a strong urge to prove themselves. If their confidence is shattered due to some event or criticism, panic and a considerable fear of failure can develop! Then *Argentum nitricum* — together with the right words — can work wonders and bring out the original zest again.

Giving confidence

Argentum nitricum children need security, and their confidence is increased just by having someone nearby! The fear can take on different shapes for them. Silver is related to the power of imagination, and in their imagination anything can happen, even if completely impossible in reality! Buildings can fall on them, trains can suddenly derail, and they can be susceptible to all sorts of illnesses. Even if they've learned very early on that a serious illness cannot be transmitted by shaking hands, they're still afraid of being infected in this way.

Most *Argentum nitricum* children suffer from claustrophobia, are afraid of crowds, and have fear of heights. These fears can really paralyze them, such that they're hindered in the development of their skills.

When *Argentum nitricum* fits the whole picture, it's able to reduce these fears to an acceptable level, and can so help these children to develop themselves as much as possible.

Physical symptoms

The complaints are concentrated on the left side of the body.

Argentum nitricum children are mostly warm-blooded and tolerate heat poorly. They love being in the fresh air, which generally does them good. Their complaints and pains are mostly worse between 09:00 and 13:00 (9 a.m. and 1 p.m.).

Argentum nitricum has a strong effect on eye infections, for which the remedy is known in conventional medicine. The throat pain corresponding to *Argentum nitricum* is very characteristic: left-sided pains worsened by swallowing and improved by cold drinks. If someone says they have the feeling of a splinter stuck in the throat, this is an additional hint that *Argentum nitricum* is the correct remedy.

The voice is the most sensitive organ. Where the strength is, there also is the weakness: as soon as these children become unsettled, it shows in their voice. The voice becomes hoarse and they can even lose their voice or begin to stutter.

The gut is sensitive and can rumble, especially with nervousness. There is frequently flatulence and diarrhea or constipation.

Food and Drink

Argentum nitricum children mostly have a strong desire for sweet things and often also for cheese. They also like fresh food and chocolate as well as salt and fat sometimes.

There can be a dislike of fat and cheese. They often also get complaints after eating sugar, fat, cabbage, pepper, and cucumbers. Their gut reacts very sensitively to these foods.

Argentum nitricum in the Clinic

Lianne

With one of my little patients, I experienced clearly how strong the effect of the remedy can be on self-confidence, and how this not only affects the child but also those around it.

It's around twelve years ago that I met Lianne, an eight-year-old girl. She had many fears and was being bullied at school. Every morning, she was afraid to go to school. Due to her anticipatory anxiety and her fear of failure, I gave her a dose of *Argentum nitricum* 30c.

Her self-confidence increased in a short time and her fears almost completely disappeared. She told me with amazement six weeks later that it was precisely the children who had been bullying her who were now ringing her doorbell in the morning and asking to go with her to school!

The Arnica montana Child

Mountain tobacco, Arnica

Plant remedy (Asteraceae family)

"I'm absolutely fine!"

Origin

Arnica grows on the mountain slopes of the Alps — and with good reason! In these dangerous areas, there is no more useful remedy than *Arnica* montana for accidents.

From time immemorial, climbers — the first to go into the mountains in spring — have plucked and chewed some *Arnica* on the way. This helps them avoid getting painful muscles the next day, as would otherwise happen. The muscle stiffness is caused by lots of tiny hemorrhages in the muscle tissue, which is not (yet) used to this type of exertion. *Arnica* apparently helps this bleeding heal more quickly.

Homeopaths know that *Arnica* has a far wider spectrum of action than this. We know many cases of people who, after a car accident with serious internal bleeding, made it to hospital where they could be operated on. It seems as if the body itself is enabled to stop the bleeding. For this reason, *Arnica* belongs to the first-aid remedies and should always be in every home medicine cabinet! Many top sportspeople use *Arnica* to recover more quickly after injuries or over-exertion.

A strong resistance

Arnica belongs to the family known as the sunflower, daisy, or aster family (Asteraceae or Compositae). In homeopathy, there are several remedies produced from this family of plants. Well-known remedies include *Bellis perennis* (common daisy) and *Millefolium* (yarrow), but the most "famous" is *Chamomilla* (true chamomile). These are well-tried "child remedies" as well as being "injury remedies."

43

The common factor with these remedies is their strong power of resistance. Children who need one of these remedies don't let on how defenseless they are. They want to give the outside world the impression that they're strong and invulnerable. *Arnica* children surpass all others at this.

This requires lots of energy, and *Arnica* children have enough of that. They're naturally very confident in their own abilities, like to be independent, and will not be reprimanded by anyone. But deep inside, there obviously remains the fear of being wounded. The façade of invulnerability is a reaction to this fear, a way of behaving that they pick up early on so as to protect themselves.

"Just don't touch me!"

This "invulnerability" comes out most strongly when an *Arnica* child is sick. They can react angrily with expressions like: "There's nothing wrong with me!" It's unimaginable for them to show their weakness. They therefore have difficulty being comforted because this reminds them that there is indeed something wrong with them. If something is troubling them, *Arnica* children want to be left in peace. They either don't react to questions or they react irritably. They have no desire to talk about their complaints.

The conventional doctor will have difficulty fathoming what is wrong with them. Homeopathic doctors, on the other hand, will recognize that these are *Arnica* children precisely due to this negative behavior, regardless of what's wrong with them! Obviously, the physical exam is nonetheless still necessary. Yet this proves to be much easier after the remedy has taken effect, since *Arnica* children normally do everything they can to avoid contact.

In general, *Arnica* children have a dislike of touch, whoever it comes from. When they don't feel well, they fear that anyone they meet will try and do something to them.

Challenging and testing

A patient told her homeopath how she had learned as a child to stand up for herself. She had noticed that her vigorous behavior — as a child this included lashing out — commanded respect. Everyone thought she was strong and powerful, although in fact she was very fearful. This behavior became her solution to deal with her inner fear.

To prove that they are "powerful," *Arnica* children need a challenge and will get themselves into fights with other children. They often win. Winning is for them a way to prove themselves, and therefore they love competition.

Self-confident on the outside

Arnica children are self-confident on the outside. They go their own way and can definitely take on leadership roles due to their charisma. So long as nothing happens to them, they feel capable of anything.

From the moment they get injured or find out in some other way how vulnerable they are physically, they become more cautious. Such an event can be so traumatic that their boisterousness flips over into fear.

Arnica can not only accelerate the healing of physical injury, but also restore the lost confidence in the child's own body.

Willpower

One of the most important character traits of *Arnica* children is their strong willpower. They want to succeed at whatever they've got into their head. On the one hand, their urge for independence plays a big role here but, on the other hand, they want to avoid at all costs being beaten. This character trait is so pronounced that they carry on until they literally "fall over." They don't allow themselves to be held back by physical complaints, which they experience as weaknesses that they don't want to show. They don't want to fail! For example, *Arnica* children with a serious cut can continue playing a hockey game right to the end; they just don't want to have anything to do with the fact that their knee is bleeding.

Accidents

Arnica has a strong relationship to accidents, and is one of the best first-aid remedies. Yet it seems as if *Arnica* children are actually drawn towards accidents — or alternatively they absolutely want to avoid them. If a child has had complaints ever since an accident,

Arnica would be the first remedy we should think of. If the "impregnable fortress" has once been violated, everything is destroyed. The comparison with Achilles comes to mind. As a newborn, he was dipped in the river Styx by his mother to make him invulnerable. To do this, she had to hold him by the ankle, which meant that this small area was left unprotected. The arrow that eventually struck him in his "Achilles heel" killed him.

Physical symptoms

Arnica is the first remedy for all after-effects of falls or blows. All injuries to do with bruising or inner bleeding heal more quickly when *Arnica* is given.

As for all remedies of the Compositae family, *Arnica* is helpful for flu, throat infections, and high fever. Less well-known for *Arnica* are the skin complaints. For boils and eczema, what stands out is that the symptoms occur symmetrically — on the same parts of the body on the right and left.

Food and Drink

Arnica children have a strong desire for sour food and drink. They have an aversion to milk and meat.

When they don't feel well, they mostly have no appetite at all. They should be given enough to drink. Going without eating for a while is usually not so bad, especially when the body itself is asking for this.

The Arsenicum album Child

White arsenic (the form used is Arsenic trioxide = As$_2$O$_3$)

Mineral remedy

"Orderly and pedantic"

Origin

This substance was discovered in the Middle Ages and was given the Greek name *"arsenikos,"* which means "masculine." It's not clear for what reason the alchemists — they were the chemists and mineral experts of their day — chose this name.

For hundreds of years, minerals containing arsenic were used as medicines, although most people immediately think of poison when they hear the name arsenic. But we need to take into account that almost all substances can heal in a specific dose, yet become poisonous in too high a dose. Just think of alcohol. Scientific investigations have proved that a glass of wine from time to time can prevent hardening of the arteries, whereas everyone knows the consequences of consuming too much alcohol!

In the introduction to the description of this remedy, Hahnemann — the founder of homeopathy — mentions the example of iron: one can produce a useful plow as well as a deadly weapon from it! As a homeopathic remedy, *Arsenicum album* is so highly dilute that it no longer has a detrimental effect. Instead, it gives the body an impulse to heal itself.

Hahnemann was not only a doctor but also a chemist. The famous chemist Berzelius, who lived at the same time, praised the outstanding chemical knowledge of Hahnemann. Before he discovered homeopathy, Hahnemann had written a comprehensive book on the effects of *Arsenicum* based on extensive research. Due to his comprehensive knowledge of languages, he was able to study Arabic and Hebrew writings. He already knew a lot about the effect of the mineral as a medicine, and the last two hundred years have shown how right he was.

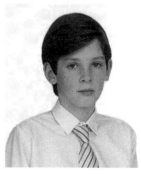

Ars.

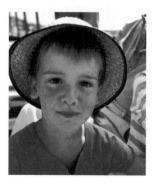

Ars.

From newborn to senior

All homeopathic remedies are suitable for every age group. In theory, there are no remedies for children or remedies for adults but practice shows that there are remedies that are prescribed more frequently for children, such as *Calcarea carbonica* and *Chamomilla*. On the other hand, some remedies — such as *Conium* — are nearly always prescribed for older people. *Arsenicum album* is an important remedy for newborns as well as for people at the end of their life.

It's prescribed more often for infants on the basis of recognizable physical symptoms, whereas at nursery school age, the character traits belonging to the remedy are already becoming clear.

Never dirty

In a group, the *Arsenicum album* children are easy to distinguish from the others. Everything about them is clean and tidy, even if they've been playing in the sandpit. They just don't get dirty!

They're extremely careful with their personal possessions, which is why they find it hard to share their toys with others. Frugality is another important characteristic. Even as youngsters, they know the value of things and love to collect pretty things. Although they often feel fearful inside, you can't always tell since they give the impression of having everything under control. Young children often betray their inner tension by nervousness and restlessness.

Arsenicum album children often suffer from eczema. After administration of this remedy, not only is the skin better, but they also become inwardly more relaxed.

Positively tidy

When they can choose their own clothes, these are very tasteful. In all weathers, their hair is immaculate, and their trousers or dress remain crease-free. The same is true of their personal things. Everything is in the right place, nothing is lying around, and everything is as new. They don't like any change, and can only rest when everything is just as they would like it. They are strong-willed and in this respect they're similar to *Nux vomica* children. This is why these two remedies are often mixed up. *Arsenicum album* children have the same perfection and staying power. However, there are clear differences and symptoms specific to this remedy.

Sulfur children also show certain similarities. The characteristic thing about *Sulfur* children is, however, that they're precise and orderly in things that interest them, but very disorderly in things that don't interest them. Their stamp collection looks perfect, but their clothes are strewn all over the floor. They can wear crease-free trousers or a crease-free dress, but forget to polish their shoes. This would never happen to an *Arsenicum album* child! If their parents don't clean their shoes, they do it themselves.

Collecting

Collecting and saving are character traits that we often find in *Arsenicum album* children. You never know what you might need later! This is also similar to *Sulfur* children. Yet *Arsenicum album* children arrange things neatly into albums, tins, or boxes. Whether it's a stamp collection, old postcards, or toy cars, they know exactly what each is worth. *Arsenicum album* children love possession, as it gives them security, and this feeling of security is for them the most important thing of all.

Worry and fear of loss

Just as they treat their things very carefully, they also treat people in their charge with the utmost care. They will do anything to maintain

49

a relationship, and to provide anything that the other person might be missing. They create their own world, their own secure environment, and do not like to see this destroyed. If they feel well inwardly and are at ease in their surroundings, they will also try to create the necessary security for others.

Deep inside is the fear of losing everything. Most of all, therefore, they like to preserve everything and to leave it as it is. Their fear relates to material things as well as to people. The biggest fear is the fear of death, of the loss of life. This fear can break out in children when someone near to them dies. The death of the grandfather or the grandmother can affect them more deeply than expected. Then *Arsenicum album* helps them to get things back into perspective. Of course, it's natural to get distressed about death and to need to work it through, yet fear — especially fear of death — can be quite paralyzing for these children.

Restless and fearful

When the fear cannot be cured, they get restless, and especially at night, when it's dark, they imagine things. They can develop many fears such as fear of thieves, of death, of an infection, of an incurable illness, and fear of being abandoned by parents or friends. Everything must be in the right place, and in their room nothing may be changed, since that also causes fear and restlessness. They try — sometimes almost obsessively — to get everything under control and so to get the upper hand over their fear. They're not always friendly towards others in such moments. They are demanding and don't seem to care what other people think or want. *Arsenicum album* children can then be mean and sarcastic. That's their way of compensating for their fears.

A small dose of this wonderful remedy helps these children to regain their equilibrium and to discover a sense of security in themselves.

Physical symptoms

Arsenicum album children freeze easily and are often quite skinny, although there are always exceptions. The complaints range from hay fever with much sneezing and watery, burning nasal discharge through eczema to serious illnesses. When they suffer from headaches, it's noticeable that they prefer cold applications, whereas in general they prefer warmth.

The skin eruptions can be very varied, from eczema to boils, with itching and burning. We generally see a worsening at night.

Watery diarrhea with shivering and restlessness is a strong indication for this remedy. Although it's a question of the whole picture, the child type, this remedy is very helpful for many acute illnesses.

Food and Drink

Arsenicum album children prefer warm food and drink, often sour and fatty, although they can also have an aversion to meat and fat. Fat and oil generally disagree with them, and many Arsenicum album children do not tolerate fruit, ice, and cold food and drink well.

A special symptom of Arsenicum album children is that they have a desire for cold water during illness, which they drink in small sips.

The Aurum metallicum Child

Gold (Au). Mineral remedy

"A heart of gold"

Origin

Gold has been known since time immemorial. This precious metal is used in almost every culture, originally for the creation of religious objects or artifacts for the rulers. In the symbolism of gold, we can already find a number of characteristics that we also see in *Aurum* children.

Gold stands for the sun, the heavenly body essential to life and, therefore, worshiped as a God by many ancient peoples. The animal that corresponds to gold in astrology is the lion, the king of the beasts. The heart is the organ symbolically related to gold, and when *Aurum* children are settled, they really do have a heart of gold!

Serious children

In newborns and young children, it's difficult to recognize the *Aurum* picture. Although the physical complaints may match, the character is only clearly recognizable after a number of years.

Aurum children are serious at an early age and need little encouragement to take on responsibility. Therefore, it's important to watch that these children in particular do not take on too much at too young an age — otherwise they'll try and take on everything! They are appreciated by children of the same age, because they like to take the initiative in exciting activities, and they know how to captivate others with their winning personality. They don't shrink from challenges, but they seldom take irresponsible risks. They are born leaders and refuse to share their position of power. If another child wants to be the leader, he or she must find another group, since *Aurum* children will not be driven out from their leadership position. When they feel it necessary, they can express their fury in an unmistakable way and will even fight for their "kingdom."

Responsibility

The sense of responsibility in *Aurum* children is strongly developed. If the family appeals to them, they will — however young they may be — attempt to meet the demands. In our clinic, we often see this development in single-parent families or when the oldest child has left. They know what they can do and are not easily destabilized, even when considerably nagged by inner doubt. Exactly like *Platina* children, they automatically assume leading positions — first in the circle of friends, then in an organization or a firm, and maybe later in a larger association. But they know that you have to work for this! Otherwise the sun won't rise; stagnation means retreat. They demand a lot, not only from themselves but also from others. They don't only do sport for fun. They want to win and won't tolerate it when others are careless and show no effort. They derive their love of life from their actions, since they know their duty and duly fulfill it. *Aurum* children are mostly serious: they're "as good as gold."

Worthy

Aurum children have something worthy of respect about them, like the lion, the king of the animals. They are conscientious, incorruptible, and do everything with full commitment. They like to always be the best, whether in sporting or academic performance. *Aurum* children like to be treated with respect. They are slow to show their emotions and, therefore, appear somewhat reserved, yet they love to be seen — just as gold will be seen to shine. They're certainly no little angels, although many *Aurum* children are drawn to religious "matters." In times of need, they can, for example, seek refuge in prayer. In general, they have high self-esteem. If something doesn't work out as they imagined, they can get really furious. It's striking that they can then shake with rage.

Sadness at failure

When everything around them is going well, *Aurum* children enjoy the good side of life. But as soon as an unforeseen problem arises or there is a problem with something for which they've taken responsibility, they get the blues. With the same intensity that they devoted themselves to something they found important, they can also make a flop of it. They experience every failure as a personal setback, and it can sometimes go so far that they feel their whole life to be worthless. *Aurum* is one of the most important remedies for sad children. If at this time they receive *Aurum*, they can reappraise the situation more easily and find the strength to start again. They may possibly then succeed in reducing their expectations!

Physical symptoms

Although we need to be careful when assigning certain external characteristics to a homeopathic type, it's very striking with *Aurum* that many children tend to be dark — with dark hair and dark eyes. Moreover, they like dressing in clean, dark clothes.

Aurum children freeze easily, yet need fresh air. They're real night owls and it's not surprising that they easily get sleep disturbances. Many complaints arise in the night at 3 a.m. — as with *Nux vomica* children, with whom they have much in common. Headaches, eye complaints, ear infections, swollen glands — almost every organ can be affected. Rheumatic complaints occur frequently with *Aurum*. One joint after the other can be swollen, with movement easing the symptoms. In boys we often see complaints of the genitals, especially the testicles.

Food and Drink

They like good food, including meat, green vegetables, bread, and milk. But there can also be an aversion to meat.

The Barium carbonicum Child

Barium carbonate (BaCO$_3$). Mineral remedy

"Growing with the right support"

Origin

Barium is a chemical element that is only found naturally in compounds with other elements. The name is derived from the Greek word *"barys,"* which translates to "heavy," and means mighty and powerful in the figurative sense. The best-known application of barium is the "barium meal," a drink given to patients in hospital before they are x-rayed in the stomach or gut. Since barium is opaque to x-rays, the digestive tract is clearly visible on the image. Moreover, barium is often used in the aerospace industry, due to its specific gravity and its opacity and air-tightness.

Missing self-confidence

Barium carbonicum children (also called *Baryta carbonica* children) are comparable to *Calcarea carbonica* children. With every new step in life, they ask themselves "Can I really do that?" or "Dare I really do that?" This, however, says nothing about their abilities. *Barium carbonicum* children can be very intelligent and can hold important posts as adults. Their challenge is to learn to cope with their self-

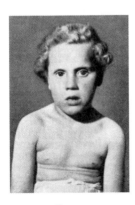

Bar-c.

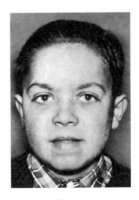

Bar-c.

55

doubt and their powerlessness, and to overcome these feelings. These children's self-confidence and belief in themselves is extremely easily upset.

At first, they hesitate with strangers and in new situations to see "how the wind blows," which is basically no bad thing. If they receive the right care, affirmation, and motivation, they can develop their inborn capabilities in the best possible way. Should an unforeseen problem arise, *Barium carbonicum* can help to get their development going again.

Inhibited development and ridicule

The *Barium carbonicum* picture is often clearly visible in children with delayed development. It can be the result of an innate handicap or, for example, due to a physical illness. Especially when they become aware that they are less capable than their playmates of the same age, problems can arise. This feeling of being "not able to do much" or of being "lesser" or "smaller" can arise from problems at school. Teasing or derogatory remarks from the teacher can trigger a *Barium carbonicum* state. Of course, these children are not actually inferior — they just feel that way. This feeling of inferiority, on the other hand, arouses negative reactions in other children. They very easily become the object of ridicule and teasing. Their self-confidence deteriorates even further, and as a result, their performance too — a vicious circle develops.

Along with appropriate behavior by the parents and teachers, *Barium carbonicum* helps these children to develop more self-confidence. As a consequence, the reactions of those around them start to change. If you respect yourself, others will also tend to respect you. Obviously, the tormentors themselves also sometimes need a homeopathic remedy, since behind the urge to torment others there is often a similar set of problems. They compensate for their lack of self-confidence by annoying others.

Cautious and stubborn

At first glance, *Barium carbonicum* children seem to be simple and docile. They're shy and they downplay their abilities so that less will be expected of them. One way of hiding their lack of self-confidence is to play the buffoon or the clown. But that's just on the surface.

They're not especially sure of themselves, and so they seem to be easily impressionable. Yet they basically know very well what they want; they just dare not express it or show it. But when they're in calm, secure, and friendly surroundings, they take the initiative, since they have willpower and even innate leadership qualities. In the family, a class, or an association, this character trait can be strengthened. Once they've taken up a clear position, they turn out to be careful and sensitive. They aren't dictatorial, although they can certainly resist if they have a different opinion.

To get used to a new situation and new people, however, they do need some time. For these children, the regular support of the parents is very important, as it's difficult for them to act independently without help.

Fear of being laughed at

When *Barium carbonicum* children are asked what they are afraid of, they often say that they're afraid of being laughed at. It's even more likely that they don't dare to say this to a strange doctor on the first visit. Therefore, it's important to talk with one or both parents about the child's character. This can usually be done without a problem in the presence of the child, but with *Barium carbonicum* children it's often better for the parents to have a quick talk with the doctor or to write down the points that are most difficult to talk about. These children are very sensitive, especially when they are being talked about. If they feel that, in their eyes, negative things are being said about them, they might possibly never want to return to this doctor.

The fear of not being taken seriously or of being laughed at sits very deep in them. If someone laughs, the child quickly has the feeling of being laughed at. If people are talking together, they mostly think that they are the subject of conversation.

On the first visit, the child might hide behind the parents or sit underneath a chair. *Barium carbonicum* children avoid direct eye-contact and do not want to be observed. We also see this behavior in *Calcarea carbonica* and *Natrium muriaticum* children.

Sluggish and clumsy

Barium carbonicum children are physically and mentally a bit clumsy. Their thinking is slow and they need time to understand things fully, which is one of the causes of their problems at school. Barium carbonicum can strengthen self-confidence in cases of inborn disability, yet in practice it repeatedly turns out that hidden talents can blossom.

The demands made of children by society are mainly of an intellectual kind, and everything should be as fast as possible. This has a detrimental effect on Barium carbonicum children. As soon as they have a little more time, they often turn out to be cleverer than suspected.

Physical symptoms

Each area of the body seems to be affected by slowness. The growth of Barium carbonicum children can be delayed or they can fail to gain weight properly. It seems as if they don't actually want to get any bigger. The defense against illness is slow to establish itself. The immune system does react, but only overcomes the illness with great difficulty. The tonsils and lymph nodes swell and harden while the children are still suffering from a chronic cold.

Their abdomen is often swollen, and their feet can sweat and smell bad. They tend to get chilly, and tolerate cold and dampness poorly. For various developmental disorders such as learning to walk and talk, but also with obesity, Barium carbonicum can be helpful.

Food and Drink

These children often have a desire for milk. They either love sweet things or have an aversion to them.

We often see a dislike of fruit, especially plums and bananas.

Barium carbonicum in the Clinic

Lucia

Lucia was retarded from birth. At the age of four, she still could not speak and her motor development was slow. She was well built and she kept her arms and legs close to her body. The main reason why her parents had come was constipation. Although she regularly had bowel movements, she could only produce small amounts and with difficulty. Generally, she was very wooden in her movements. She had difficulty bending and was very stiff when running.

She was shy, fearful, and slow, very cautious and self-controlled. Even as a newborn baby, she was afraid of strangers and her development proceeded in very small steps. Yet when she was occupied with something, she could play for a long time with great concentration and was very exact. She didn't know, however, how to behave when she had the choice between two things. This completely bewildered her. She could only concentrate on one thing at a time. When she wanted something, she was extremely stubborn. Otherwise, she tried to avoid any attention and when people looked at her, she made herself as small as possible.

First, I prescribed her *Calcarea carbonica*. Although there was some improvement, she remained stiff and wooden. Only when she received *Barium carbonicum*, first 30c then later 200c and 1,000c (1M), did things gradually start to look up for her, and she caught up slowly but surely in all areas.

At school, where she received special tutoring, things went very well. Her speech got better and better, and she became freer in her behavior. Her movements were more fluid, her balance improved, and she felt capable of taking on more. *Barium carbonicum* saw to it that she felt better.

Bastian

Bastian was five when I first saw him. His complaints, for which his mother had sought my help, were regularly recurring colds, enlarged tonsils, and difficulty speaking.

The way he behaved during the first consultation was characteristic for the remedy. Bastian was initially very shy — as soon as I looked at

59

him, he turned his head away and tried to hide behind his mother. His mother said that he had developed normally since birth but was rather slow at learning to talk and also did not speak clearly. He often let his tongue hang out of his mouth and was unmistakably knock-kneed.

Bastian regularly had a cold with fever and coughing. When he was ill, he felt very tired and coughed up green mucus. The family doctor prescribed a course of antibiotics each time, and the ear, nose, and throat specialist had already removed his adenoids, but none of this had helped very much.

Bastian was always very hungry and craved sweet things and fruit. He didn't like unusual foods, especially beans. He slept well; in the evening he himself asked if he could go to bed, although for a long time he had slept with his parents in their bed.

He was a curious and smart boy who could, nevertheless, also be very unsettled and fearful. He couldn't be without his mother. He was strong-willed and he liked to play the boss, including with his older brother. In general, he was affectionate and clingy — he sat on his mother's lap and liked to be pampered — but he could also get very furious. His sensitivity to criticism was obvious. He quickly got the feeling of being laughed at.

I saw him again six weeks after the first dose of *Barium carbonicum* 30c. He had had one more cold, but this time the cold had cleared up on its own. He was more energetic, calmer, better able to concentrate, and his self-confidence was significantly better.

I prescribed him *Barium carbonicum* 200c and didn't see him again until a year later. In the winter, he had had one more cold, but this had cleared up without medication. Otherwise Bastian was very well. He felt happy and was full of self-confidence. He was still a bit slow at everything.

When he had ear trouble, this disappeared after a dose of *Barium carbonicum* 1,000c (1M). Six months later, his mother called to tell me that Bastian was still doing well. At school, they were pleased with his concentration and the pace of his work.

The Belladonna Child

Deadly nightshade, Dwale, Banewort, Devil's cherries, Naughty man's cherries, Divale, Black cherry, Devil's herb, Great morel, Dwayberry

Plant remedy

(Solanaceae family = Nightshades)

"Intense will to live"

Origin

Atropa belladonna is the Latin name of the plant known as "deadly nightshade." It's an herbaceous plant that grows to 2-5 feet (50-150 cm) high with green leaves, violet or brown flowers, and in the mature state it has shiny black berries. The plant blooms between June and August.

Its name comes from the Greek *"atropos"* ("the inevitable"), which refers to one of the three fateful goddesses whose task it is to cut the thread of life. Without a doubt, this is connected to the great toxicity of these attractive berries, as expressed in the name "Deadly Nightshade." Yet the name has another meaning, since *Belladonna* has protected many people from death: *"Bella donna"* translates to "beautiful woman" and refers to the fact that women used to trickle the juice into their eyes to dilate their pupils and so increase

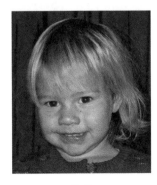

Bell.

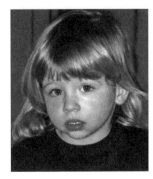

Bell.

61

their beauty. The pupils then looked exactly like the black berries of this plant. Atropine, one of the active substances, is still used today in ophthalmology to dilate the pupils for examination. *Belladonna* is also used in conventional medicine for intestinal cramps.

Unbridled natural forces

Belladonna children have a strong force in them. For parents and teachers, it's a major and not always easy challenge to direct this energy into the right channels.

All the emotions of *Belladonna* children are vehement and intense. They show their feelings directly and uninhibitedly. When they are happy, they're beside themselves with joy. When they speak, they do it so loudly that everyone can hear. And woe betide you if they're angry ...

Elisabeth Kübler-Ross has written that anger lasts only 15 seconds in children, and that it's very important to let them have these 15 seconds before intervening. This is not always easy since most grown-ups are conditioned to react immediately. Almost everyone has the idea that anger shouldn't be allowed.

For *Belladonna* children, it's all the more important to let them experience their anger, since the underlying forces are so strong. Immediate intervention causes the anger to be directed inwards, only to emerge all the more violently later on.

Vehement and intense

Atropa belladonna belongs to the Solanaceae (nightshade) family. These plants harbor the dark powers of the night, but the Latin name also contains the word *"sol,"* which means *"sun"*. All nightshades wrestle with the dilemma of how to positively use their enormous powers so that they don't have to shy away from the light of day. Their emotions — such as vehement passion, fear, and fury — are intense and almost brutish.

Belladonna children have many similarities with *Tuberculinum* children. Life seems too short and they want to experience so much. Both child types are very unsettled and grind their teeth at night. They want to grab hold of everything that attracts their attention. They want to literally "grasp" life. *Belladonna* children are even more vehement in their emotional reactions. If they're really furious, which can easily happen, they'll do anything to be rid of the fury: kick, hit, scream, and even bite. At such moments they are unreachable and simply cannot be brought to their senses.

Hyperactive

Belladonna is a typical remedy for children. Yet this doesn't mean that we only prescribe it for children. There are also adults for whom this picture still fits. Their way of reacting has something childlike: direct and uninhibited. The emotions are much stronger than we suppose. In the course of their lives, these adults have learned to control themselves because, like the children, they know what the reaction of the outside world will be if they lose control. For this reason, children can be very obedient in school but exactly the opposite at home, similar to *Anacardium* ("at school an angel, at home a rascal"). The fits of rage shown by *Belladonna* children are, however, much stronger. When the emotions get the upper hand, this can result in hyperactivity and even Attention-Deficit Hyperactivity Disorder (ADHD). The child suffers from unimaginable inner agitation that is hard to handle, resulting in fits of rage and uncontrolled behavior.

Together with *Lithium phosphoricum*, *Tuberculinum*, and *Stramonium*, *Belladonna* belongs to the remedies that are able to restore balance in hyperactive children.

Fight or flight

When *Belladonna* children meet with resistance, they start fighting. "Bella" is the Latin plural of "bellum," which means "war." Fight or flight. The deep fear that drives them is the fear of death. They want to live!

We also see this picture when they're ill. With an infection or during flu, they always react very violently with high fever and immense heat. The body takes the fight straight to the enemy. During an attack of fever, *Belladonna* children often have terrifying visions. Fever with delirium and confused speech is typical for this remedy picture. Apart from that, these children have few fears. In the healthy state, they are very strong and can put up a good fight. One of the few unmistakable fears is the fear of dogs (exactly as for

Tuberculinum and *Lycopodium*). Possibly this relates to the "wolf" in them. *Belladonna* is also called "Devil´s cherries" (*"Wolfskirsche"*) in German, just as *Lycopodium* is called "wolfpaw"!

Only when they realize the fight is hopeless do they flee. Children with high fever can want to flee the room due to fear of imaginary monsters or other frightening images.

Physical symptoms

Fever, headache, and a sensitive nervous system are the most important symptoms of *Belladonna*. Anyone with flu or an infection can go into a *Belladonna* state, but experience shows that this acute picture occurs particularly often in *Calcium carbonicum* children.

Furthermore, a typical characteristic is sudden fever. A child can be playing peacefully, and just a quarter of an hour later be lying deliriously, even with febrile seizures. *Belladonna* can prevent such febrile seizures when given at the right time. With fever, the head is glowing hot, whereas the hands and feet feel cold. The color of the face — fiery red with glistening eyes, dilated pupils, and visibly pulsating blood vessels in the neck — resembles the picture that the berries cause in cases of poisoning. During an attack of fever, they can look hounded, and they can hallucinate. Children see monsters or mysterious faces and it's almost impossible to talk to them in this, for them, unaccustomed state of fear.

With *Belladonna*, the complaints are mostly on the right, for throat as well as for ear infections. The *Belladonna* picture could also fit an acute appendicitis. Obviously the child must then be admitted straight to hospital.

Belladonna is very important for the treatment of headaches. Here again, it is true that children of different constitutional types can be helped acutely with their headaches, not only *Belladonna*-type children. The headache might be caused, for example, by chilling of the head following a haircut, or also by overheating following exposure to the sun. The pain, which can be awful for the child, is worsened by the slightest movement or jolt. The child wants complete rest without any light at all. Warmth mostly soothes. When in addition the head is bright red and hot, while the hands and feet feel cold, the decision to go for *Belladonna* is clear!

Food and Drink

Belladonna children ask for lemonade, lemons, and bread. They dislike water, acidic things, warm food, and coffee, as well as vegetables, soups, and fat.

Belladonna in the Clinic

Marlies

Marlies was just four years old when I saw her for the first time. She had had problems since birth, cried often, and grew slowly. After several months, she was admitted to hospital with bronchitis-like symptoms. Afterwards, she always had a cold, picked up fevers quickly, and regularly had ear infections.

When she was one year old, she had her first fever convulsion. Since these convulsions kept recurring, the pediatrician prescribed various anti-epilepsy drugs — yet without success.

Marlies was a sociable child, but was also very stubborn. She would never do anything that she didn't want to, and any form of compulsion only had the opposite effect. She loved movement, liked climbing, and liked to be in the open most of all. When things didn't go as she wanted, she threw herself on the floor and bit, hit, and screamed.

Due to the febrile seizures, I gave her a dose of *Belladonna*, to which she reacted very well. The improvement occurred not only on the physical plane, but also in her behavior. From time to time, she still caught a cold, which healed on its own, but the febrile seizures stopped. Marlies listened more to her parents, had fewer fits of rage, and generally became friendlier.

The Beryllium metallicum Child

Beryllium (Be). Mineral remedy

"What do they think of me?"

Origin

Our earth consists of many solid elements. The best known are silicium (sand, flint or quartz), carbon (graphite), and metals such as aluminum and iron. The metal beryllium is less well-known, but is at least as important as a homeopathic remedy.

After lithium, beryllium is the lightest solid substance on earth. As the name clearly indicates, beryllium occurs in the precious stone beryl. This name apparently comes from Berul, a city in Iraq. A further explanation for the name of this element is the Greek term "berullos," which means "sea-green." Beryl was used in the past for the production of glasses — hence the German name for glasses (spectacles), *"Brille"*!

Apart from in the colorless to white mineral beryl, beryllium also occurs in other types of rock. Beryllium salts taste sweet, which is why beryllium is sometimes called glucinium (from glucose). Together with transparency and hardness — it's harder than steel — beryllium has some other characteristics that explain the homeopathic effect. It's very elastic, which is why it's used in alloys for the production of springs.

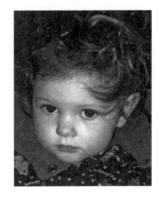

Beryl-c.

Seen through someone else's glasses

Children who need *Beryllium* tend to see themselves as if through someone else's glasses. We find this character trait in various remedies, of which *Calcarea carbonica* is the most famous. There's a feeling of uncertainty about oneself and the need for recognition from

67

the other person. *Beryllium* children doubt whether they can simply be as they are. They find criticism difficult to bear. Due to the conditions in which they grew up, they were unable to develop self-respect and self-esteem. They feel as if they're "transparent," vulnerable, and unsure. They don't have the courage to make their own decisions or to confront conflicts, which is similar to *Thuja* children. They haven't learned to take on relationships, and even have trouble sensing what they want or who they really are. They look for this outside themselves, in someone who they think is stronger than they are.

Adaptation and hiding

What do the others think of me? To find recognition, they tend to adapt themselves and become subordinate to others. The ability to empathize and the desire for recognition make them ideal helpers. This may be what helps them to justify their existence. Yet this adaptation can cause them to become a stranger to themselves, which in turn leads them to behave in a passive and uncertain way, so that other people end up making decisions for them. This further weakens their feeling of self-esteem, since they never show who they really are. The way that others treat them can even give them the feeling of being "bad."

Once they have this feeling, they tend to hide themselves and to be inconspicuous. Shame and self-criticism can start to play a big role. It can even go so far that they withdraw from reality. They are physically present, but feel helpless and powerless inside.

Self-Love

The problem for *Beryllium* children is really not so much what other people think of them, but more their verdict on themselves. They lack a foundation of trust. While *Silicium, Natrium muriaticum,* or *Sulfur* children can't tolerate the idea that the other person does not love them, *Beryllium* children have difficulty loving themselves.

The picture of *Beryllium* is similar to *Calcarea carbonica, Carcinosinum, Lac caninum, Borax,* and *Thuja.* The differences are subtle, and in some cases the homeopathic practitioner will have to alternate the remedies according to the symptoms displayed. *Beryllium* helps these children to sort themselves out, so that they can be themselves and love themselves in a healthy way.

Physical symptoms

Our posture betrays our inner feelings. These children tend to go through life stooped and with rounded shoulders — a sign of their lack of self-confidence. A further characteristic is that they often sit cross-legged, which could indicate that they want to defend themselves.

Mostly we see a lack of energy. The growth and development of the sexual characteristics can be delayed in *Beryllium* children, as for *Calcarea carbonica* and *Barium carbonicum* children. The same as for these two child types, *Beryllium* children also often suffer from dry skin, dry mucous membranes, and swollen glands in the neck, armpit, and groin. Moreover, they often have a dry and blocked nose, especially in the morning, as well as nose-bleeds and complaints of the airways. As with the other "major" child remedies, it's generally possible for all the organs to be affected, such as stomach, gut, kidneys, and urinary tract.

The bone complaints, which remind us greatly of *Calcium*, are striking. The bones can, for example, be too "flexible," which fits well with the overall picture of *Beryllium metallicum*.

Food and Drink

In general, they feel better for eating and drinking. Milk can cause irritation in the nose. Pancakes (made with egg) can bring on nausea and vomiting.

The Borax veneta Child

Borax, Sodium tetraborate (Na$_2$B$_4$O$_7$). Mineral remedy

"Searching for my own identity"

Origin

Borax is a salt that occurs in the mountain lakes of Tibet. The Tibetans use borax like salt to flavor their "tsampa," a kind of millet porridge, which is a basic foodstuff in this inhospitable land. The Venetians — Marco Polo visited Tibet eight hundred years ago — introduced this salt to Europe, hence the suffix "veneta" (Venetian). Dutch traders processed the raw material into useful borax, which was already being used hundreds of years ago for rashes of the mouth. Since the Dutch kept their processing method secret, the French looked for other sources of borax, and found it in some of the hot springs in Italy.

The most important element in this salt is boron, which has recently been introduced into homeopathy in the pure form. *Borax* was proved by Hahnemann and recognized as a homeopathic remedy.

Developmental phase: who am I?

Borax is a salt consisting of two chemical elements: sodium and boron, plus oxygen. The influence of boron on the homeopathic picture is considerable and a quick sketch of this element will make the picture of *Borax* clearer.

The homeopathic remedy *Borium metallicum* fits the developmental stage in which the child becomes aware of its own identity, its own "I." The age at which this occurs is around the fourth or fifth year. Children begin to understand that they are independent individuals. If something very drastic occurs in this period of life, it can restrict the development of a personal identity.

Before children enter this phase, they ideally feel themselves connected to everything and everyone in a natural way.

70

Not getting any bigger

Borax children need rest and they don't want to grow. For unknown reasons, they develop a resistance to this phase. The children defend themselves against growing up, against no longer being a child. Yet they have fewer problems with their identity than *Beryllium* children. Most of all, they want to be back in the peaceful, harmonious phase before the birth and to retain the warm connection with the mother. The peace and harmony they are seeking reminds us of the quietness of the Tibetan mountain lakes.

Quiet, please!

Every change disturbs the calm that these children are looking for. Newborns who need *Borax* cry as soon as they're put down, for example, to have their nappies (diapers) changed. The downward movement evidently makes them afraid. With older children, we also see this sensitivity to downward movement — they can't stand taking the elevator down!

Borax children are also very sensitive to other disturbances of the peace, such as sudden noises and unexpected movements. Their reactions are intense: fury, fear, and loud crying. Most of all, they want to cling to their mother or another person they trust. They obviously won't let themselves be touched by strangers.

Adapting

The *Borax* picture is different for bigger children. They would still really like to cling to someone, but that's no longer appropriate at this age. If this picture is caused by a disturbance in the process of individualization — for example, incest, abuse, or neglect — they tend to orient themselves too much to the outside world. They have no identity of their own, but behave as they're expected to and adapt themselves as well as possible. In this respect, they're similar to *Thuja* children. They're just as sensitive and empathetic, and can also retreat completely into their own world. Yet there are certain characteristics that help us to differentiate between the two remedies. While *Borax* children are very sensitive to noise — even someone biting an apple can irritate them dreadfully — *Thuja* children generally react strongly to music and are easily plagued by feelings

71

of guilt. A further difference is the fear of infection that *Borax* children can have. This is why they wash their hands so often, although they don't really like doing this!

Doubting and splitting off

Children who don't know who they really are quickly develop self-doubt. If they have to choose something, this puts them in a dreadful dilemma: "What do I really want?" At the same time, they are very disturbed by others who are unclear or have doubts. We often see a similar pattern, even in ourselves: we get most annoyed about the characteristics in others that we reject in ourselves!

Due to the difficulty in making their own decisions, they unintentionally reinforce their dependence on others.

The disturbance in the development of identity can go so far that parts get split off and, so to speak, multiple personalities develop. But this occurs only with serious traumatic events, and then only at an age in which there hasn't been a chance to develop strong self-confidence. *Borax* can help these children early on to assimilate the trauma and develop their own identity. At an advanced age, it can certainly work supportively and — together with the right therapy — maybe also heal.

Physical symptoms

Borax is one of the most important remedies for newborns with anemia. The ingestion of food is often a problem for these newborns, and the thrush that they frequently have is not exactly appetizing!

The aversion to downward movement mentioned above can lead to dizziness and even unconsciousness. In general, the organ of equilibrium is their weak spot.

The withdrawal behavior expresses itself on the physical level in the eyelids: with infections, there is often an inward movement of the eyelashes (trichiasis). The edges of the eyelids can also turn inwards (entropium).

Nutrition and digestion often cause difficulties, just as the children have difficulty digesting everyday experiences. The mucous membranes of the entire gastrointestinal tract, from the mouth to the anus, are very fragile. Eczema can occur anywhere, usually very painful white spots, often also ulcers, although these complaints usually occur in the mouth. In addition, the children often suffer from an excess flow of saliva, cracks in the tongue, nausea, vomiting, and diarrhea. Another weak spot is the bladder.

In general, *Borax* children are irritable and even tearful before they go to the bathroom. After urination or defecation, they're visibly relieved. Then they're happy and cheerful. They also feel better after they've cried or coughed something up. They have to get rid of the "rubbish," and so they suffer until they've got it out.

They recover during a walk in the fresh air. On the other hand, they can tolerate neither cold nor warmth particularly well. Tangled hair is a symptom that we often notice in *Borax* children.

Food and Drink

Borax children love apples, but they tolerate fruit badly, and also salty and sweet foods. It's typical for them to get diarrhea due to cigarette smoke. Maybe this will prevent them from picking up this unhealthy habit!

The Calcarea carbonica Child

Calcium carbonate, Oyster shell (CaCO$_3$). Mineral remedy

"Externally robust, internally vulnerable"

Origin

Calcarea carbonica is one of the most important child remedies. Traditionally, *Calcarea carbonica* was considered such a common remedy for children that approximately 40% of all children were given it at some point. However, this percentage has gone down, now that homeopaths can identify remedies such as *Lithium*, *Beryllium*, and *Boron* in children who formerly might have been given *Calcarea carbonica*. Homeopaths can now find the correct remedy for each child with greater precision.

Calcarea carbonica is not the familiar calcium we know from limestone or the scale in a water boiler, but is instead the calcium of the oyster shell. The theme of the oyster runs through the entire remedy picture.

Leaving the shell

The remedy is especially suited to the time when the child has to master the transition from the protected world of the home to the

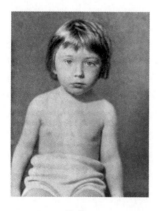
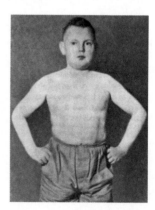

Calc-c.   *Calc-c.*

big bad outside world," for example, after kindergarten or when starting elementary school. If there are problems at this time, the remedy can help to cope with the transition. *Calcarea carbonica* strengthens the child's resolve to take the crucial steps. In the image of the oyster, the child is thereby leaving the "shell."

When such a transition causes physical complaints such as chronic colds or eczema, or delays in physical or mental development, *Calcarea carbonica* can be helpful. When we ask how the child is feeling, the parents will tell us about the difficulty the child is having with the new situation, such as a new teacher, a move, or a change from one group to the next.

See which way the wind is blowing

The characteristic *Calcarea carbonica* child has a heavy build and sweats easily on the head. Yet we also sometimes see tall and skinny children of this type. They are often late to walk and their teething is usually slower and more difficult than for other children.

The homeopath can sometimes see the picture the moment the child comes into the consulting room. These children keep a certain distance at first and prefer to sit on the lap of their father or mother. They want to see which way the wind is blowing and only say what is necessary. They are mostly quiet children who don't want to stand out.

At school, they're well-behaved and do their best in order to achieve as much as possible, not out of ambition but because they want to stay in the teacher's good graces. They are mostly attentive pupils who nevertheless need much time to assimilate the material. They fall behind their classmates, not so much due to their abilities but rather due to their pace. They work steadily, plodding along with unimaginable staying power. Once they've understood something, they never forget it afterwards. They're discouraged by too high a pace or excessive demands. Then their self-confidence declines and they lose heart. Every decisive change can throw them off balance — a dose of *Calcarea carbonica* restores the balance once more.

Childhood fears

Calcarea carbonica displays the typical childhood fears such as fear of the dark, fear of being alone, fear of heights, and fear of new things.

Anything to do with uncertainty can generate anxiety. Horror films or ghost stories disturb their sleep, because they continue to think and dream of them.

Calcarea carbonica children have a very strong will. When they don't agree with something, they show it, but mostly by stubbornness rather than rage.

Security

Security is absolutely necessary for these children. *Calcarea carbonica* children need the certainty of being able to lean on something. They must be "standing on firm ground." They are, therefore, seldom quick in their development — every new step is carefully prepared and considered. And it's not surprising that fear of heights occurs for this child type, since they prefer to be standing on firm ground. They like to know where they are. They can be worried about the future because the future means uncertainty. "What will happen ...?"

Calcarea carbonica children are known for their difficult-to-answer questions on the meaning of life and the universe. They want to know, for example, how the world came into being or where we go when we die. Their will to learn comes from their need for clarity and security.

Hard shell, soft core

Externally, these children can appear robust and powerful, but inside they are very sensitive and, therefore, vulnerable. They have trouble tolerating a negative atmosphere and have difficulty getting bad events shown on television out of their head. They prefer to have nothing to do with such things, since they remind them of how insecure life is and all the things that could happen to them. When they're feeling threatened or fearful, they "shut down" and with-draw like an oyster. This doesn't mean that they can't defend them-selves, but they only get really angry when there is no other way.

They say they find it especially hard to defend themselves against the gaze of other people. To be looked at, especially by a stranger, is always unpleasant for them. They think that people can tell when they're not feeling well, which is connected to their sensitivity to criticism. They're very sensitive to the opinions of others and, there-fore, show as much consideration as possible. They proceed cau-tiously and are always asking whether they will be able to manage everything.

The great thing about this remedy, apart from the fact that it stimu-lates the healing of the physical complaints, is that it strengthens the children internally and helps them to regain their self-confidence.

Physical symptoms

In the human body, calcium plays a very important role. Just as with the oyster, it gives us form and stability. Our skeleton and our teeth consist mostly of calcium. Calcium is essential for vari-ous functional processes in the body. Complaints that fit *Calcarea carbonica* are generally characterized by weakness. This affects not just muscles and bones but also the immune system and mental resistance. It looks as if stability is completely missing. On the other hand, hardenings and swellings can develop, as if the body is taking up too much calcium.

The physical complaints of these children mostly have to do with their resistance. When they're weakened, they get colds easily — as if they were collecting all the viruses and bacteria from their envi-ronment. If this condition intensifies, ear infections, bronchitis, or asthma can develop.

Problems with teeth and bones often indicate *Calcarea carbonica*. Even children suffering from osteogenesis imperfecta, a severe hereditary disease in which the bones are extremely brittle, can be significantly helped by *Calcarea carbonica*.

In addition, skin conditions such as eczema, warts, and calluses can occur. The glands swell very easily in these children, and they sweat more than average, both on particular parts of the body and in general.

The bones can be fragile or have abnormal growths (exostoses). Symptoms similar to those of rickets — which is softening of the bones — are typical for *Calcarea carbonica*, as is delayed closure of the fontanels or curvature of the spine. When *Calcarea carbonica* is given in time, it can prevent many of these illnesses!

Food and Drink

Very characteristic for *Calcarea carbonica* children is the strong desire for (softboiled) eggs. In the picture of the egg, we can see similarities to the oyster — the hard shell and the soft insides! Small children have a desire for indigestible things such as chalk, earth, clay, and the like, as if they want to compensate for a lack of calcium. Other beloved foodstuffs are milk and nuts — each containing calcium — and olives, salt, sweet things, and ice cream.

They have an aversion to slimy foods and fat.

There can also be an aversion to milk and they often can't tolerate it. Many complaints can be worsened by milk or be caused by milk in the first place.

Calcarea carbonica in the Clinic

Bernd

Bernd was almost ten years old when he came to me for the first time with his mother. Since his second year, he had been suffering from anemia, apprehensiveness, stomach aches, and nightmares, for which he had taken many different medications. Especially in autumn and winter everything got worse. His mother described him as a lovable, rather slow youngster who had difficulties with new situations. At school he soon got the idea that the other children were "better" than him, although he was perfectly able to learn properly. He might need a bit more time than the others, but what he learned he also mastered! Nevertheless, his self-confidence was very poor. Even when he was occasionally annoyed, he did not easily get angry. The whole story fitted the *Calcarea carbonica* picture well. I prescribed him a dose of *Calcarea carbonica* 30c. After six weeks, the shortness of breath improved for a few weeks and the stomach aches disappeared. He also looked much better, was more active, and had more self-confidence. It was noticeable that he was sweating less. Beforehand, he had been very sweaty, especially on the head during sleep. After a dose of 200c, his complaints improved some more and for longer. Later he needed a dose of 1,000c (1M) again and two doses of 10,000c (10M).

One year after the first consultation, his mother phoned to say that almost all his complaints had disappeared, and that he generally felt better. He felt shortness of breath from time to time, but this disappeared very quickly each time after a dose of *Calcarea carbonica* 10,000c (10M).

79

The Calcarea phosphorica Child

Calcium phosphate, $Ca_3(PO_4)_2$. Mineral remedy

"Friends are the foundation"

Origin

This homeopathic remedy is prepared from calcium and phosphorus, two chemical elements that are also used as individual homeopathic remedies. To produce Calcium phosphate, phosphoric acid is trickled into lime water.

Calcium phosphate plays an important role in the construction of the skeleton. Problems with the building of bone and teeth structure as well as with the healing of bone fractures can be cured with this homeopathic remedy. Since growth and the building of bone structure mainly occurs in the early years, this remedy is often prescribed for children.

In the picture of *Calcarea phosphorica*, we find symptoms that we recognize from *Calcarea carbonica* and *Phosphorus*. In the clinic, *Calcarea carbonica* is more frequently prescribed for younger children, *Calcarea phosphorica* for older children, and *Phosphorus* in the period when the children are leaving school. Yet the constitutional picture doesn't depend on age: we find it in newborn babies as well as in adults into old age.

Friendship and learning

Calcarea phosphorica children are naturally open and get to know people quickly. They are curious, love new challenges, and like to travel very much. In contrast to *Phosphorus* children, *Calcarea phosphorica* children are somewhat more reserved. This is connected to their sensitivity about what others think of them. They want to make a good impression

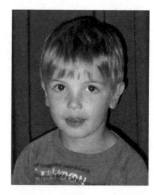

Calc-p.

80

and are therefore very sensitive to criticism, in which they resemble *Calcarea carbonica* children. A major difference to *Calcarea carbonica* is that they actually like change. They have a distaste for everyday routine. They're always searching for something new to tempt them. They are eager to learn and have an exceptionally strong need for friends. Their strength — but also their weakness — lies in learning and friendship. When everything is going well at school and they have good friends, they thrive, but when something goes wrong, problems can arise.

Difficulties at school

The demands on young children are considerable: the expectations made of four-year-olds are great, although many are not up to these expectations. There are large individual differences as far as maturity goes. Many four-year-olds are able to learn reading, writing, and arithmetic, whereas others are still playful and would rather remain a child for a while longer. Still others need time to get used to the process of learning. They already have the will and know the basics, yet they need approval every step of the way. *Calcarea phosphorica* is an important remedy for this last-mentioned group of children.

Teachers who can accurately estimate the appropriate demands to make on the children won't cause problems, but sometimes teachers sadly lack the time to give each child the attention it needs. Positive motivation gets the best from every child (and generally from every person), yet unfortunately most adults grew up with criticism and discouraging remarks. Once these children get the idea that they're not good at learning, then there's a strong chance that they will not achieve their potential, simply from fear of making mistakes. *Calcarea phosphorica* children can quickly get the feeling that they're stupid, sometimes just due to small things or passing comments. The sad thing is that this feeling can last an entire lifetime if it's not noticed and corrected. Even as adults, they can still be afraid of being perceived as "stupid."

Difficulties in concentration

The first reaction of *Calcarea phosphorica* children to criticism is that they must make more effort. They then work harder and need more time to finish their work. Out of fear of making mistakes, they become cautious and spend more time thinking. If they still can't achieve what they set out to do or don't receive the necessary approval, their self-confidence sinks. This leads them to avoid school, especially during exams, when they have to prove themselves. Lack of self-confidence saps their energy. Due to tension, they become tired more quickly and their concentration gets worse. In this phase, we find that the children suffer from headaches. Headaches in school children can be a strong indication for *Calcarea phosphorica*.

Friends

Calcarea phosphorica children have the same sensitivity towards friends. They desperately want to belong and have one or more good friends. If this doesn't work out, or if they're rejected, their self-confidence is dealt a serious blow. They can also be thrown off course by a move, a change of school, or some other event in which they lose their friends. Friends are their grounding and their security; without friends, they feel lost. A good friendship can help them through very difficult times, such as a separation or the loss of a parent.

Calcarea phosphorica helps these children to develop more self-confidence, so that they're more independent of the opinions of others, of their school performance, or of missing friends.

Physical symptoms

The remedy has a strong affinity for bones and teeth, and can improve or even heal many different complaints, such as retarded or accelerated growth, growing pains, malformations, or a delayed closing of the fontanels. The same is true of problems with the teeth, learning to walk, even through emotional development. Since phosphorus plays an important role in our thinking, *Calcarea phosphorica* can help with concentration problems and learning difficulties.

Calcarea phosphorica children feel chilly easily and like it warm. *Calcarea phosphorica* is the most important remedy for children with headaches, which are mostly the result of intellectual over-exertion.

The tonsils are frequently swollen. If the children's resistance is poor, they easily catch cold and get upper respiratory infections as well as swollen glands in the neck. Instead of removing the tonsils, it would be better to first prescribe a dose of *Calcarea phosphorica* — obviously only when the overall picture matches. We can then see how the glands go down, resistance increases, mood improves, and self-confidence rises.

Food and Drink

When newborn babies reject the mother's milk, this is possibly a suitable remedy. *Calcarea phosphorica* children prefer spicy, smoked foods, salt, fish, sweet things, and cold drinks. Yet they can sometimes have an aversion to fish and salt.

The Calcarea silicata Child

Calcium silicate (Ca₂SiO₄). Mineral remedy

"The family is the foundation"

Origin

Calcium and silicium are two important elements for the construction of the skeleton. Calcium does not occur in nature in the pure form and would anyway be too brittle, whereas pure silicium — such as quartz — would be too hard and inflexible. In the right proportions with other elements such as phosphorus, manganese, and fluoride, our bones are strong and flexible enough. When we learn about the mode of action of all elements, this enables us to better understand the effects on the physical and emotional level.

Limestone (calcium) and sand (silicium) are also the basic materials for building houses. Together with aluminum oxide, these form the hardened cement. In this way, our houses attain their final form and stability. The "house" represents not just the physical shelter, but also the family in which we grow up. Think of the term the "House of Windsor" — used to describe the modern British monarchy — which refers to the family itself rather than the bricks and mortar.

Calcarea silicata is connected not only with the reliability of the family, but also with the stability of our physical body. If something is missing here, *Calcarea silicata* as a homeopathic remedy can give the necessary boost to restore balance and stability.

What do they think of me?

Expressions such as: "He comes from a good family" indicate the influence of the family on a person's appearance. We're also formed by the people who are our role models, especially in the early years. *Calcarea silicata* children are tactful and often delicately built. They're very sensitive to the opinions of others and also to their surroundings. They're constantly aware of what others think of them, not just when they're being looked at. Since they want to make a

84

good impression, they tend to conform. Their sensitivity sometimes goes so far that they're not only aware of the people who are actually present — they can also even sense family members who have already died. *Calcarea silicata* children can, for example, see their dead grandfather sitting in his familiar armchair in their grandmother's house and can describe him in great detail. Whether this is a real apparition or the result of an over-vivid imagination is hard to judge. It's important for the child that this perception is taken seriously and not simply denied, since otherwise the child's self-confidence is damaged.

Being good and giving their best

To do justice to the picture that others have of them, these children give their best in all areas. At school, they work hard and their *Silicium* side is responsible for their exactness and precision. The father's opinion is very important to them and they directly feel his approval or disapproval, verbally as well as nonverbally!

Their self-confidence is largely dependent on the opinion of those around them. It's not as if they themselves do not know what they want or think, but they subordinate their opinion to the opinion of others.

In the world outside the family, they're sensitive to the opinion that others have of their family. "If you hurt my father, you also hurt me!" is a fitting expression for these children. Therefore, they try to be on their best behavior. Negative remarks about family members can really hurt and upset them. Yet they don't generally react immediately. Since *Calcarea silicata* children are usually rather modest and shy, they tend to withdraw.

Submissive or stubborn

As long as they give way without damaging themselves, everything's OK. But when they go too far, two things can happen: they no longer listen to themselves and become fully dependent on the opinions of others or they withdraw into stubbornness and inaction: "If you don't like what I do, I'm going on strike!" This is their inner hardness as opposed to their soft outer appearance. When their self-confidence is constantly shattered — for example, due to over-critical parents or teachers — then they miss a solid basis in their life. The idea that they can do nothing right becomes entrenched. They see criticism everywhere and become completely lacking in self-confidence. This naturally undermines their vitality and their love of life. These children appear passive and apathetic, without sufficient energy and liveliness. *Calcarea silicata* can help such children to develop a positive self image.

Physical symptoms

Lack of energy is one of the most striking symptoms of *Calcarea silicata* children who become unsettled. Their already slight bodies become thinner, sensitive to the cold, and weak. Any kind of cold worsens their condition, and they sweat on the slightest exertion, especially at the back of the head and on the hands. Night sweats and foul-smelling, sweaty feet also occur frequently. They react sensitively to the phases of the moon and particularly feel worse at full moon. Complaints often arise following immunization. Warmth and massage are mostly good for them.

Their body is susceptible to every kind of inflammation such as colds, ear infections, swollen glands, and so on. Skin inflammations can lead to pimples and even to large abscesses with a yellow, stinking discharge.

Their teeth and bones are often unhealthy, as are their skin, hair, and nails. The skin is dry, and various discharges can appear. The nails often grow inwards and become brittle or discolored.

Food and Drink

Exactly like *Calcarea carbonica* and *Silicea* children, they really go for eggs. In addition, they love salt and sweet things. They also like dishes such as pizza and lasagna. They either like or dislike milk. They can often tolerate neither milk nor fat.

The Calcarea sulfurica Child

Calcium sulfate (CaSO₄). Mineral remedy

"Do you really love me?"

Origin

The best known compound of calcium and sulfur is plaster, which is used, for example, in the building industry and also in art. Calcium gives stability, which is why it's the basis of the skeleton in the body. *Calcarea sulfurica* used to be relatively unknown as a remedy, until we developed a deeper understanding of the minerals in recent years. *Calcarea* (calcium) and *Sulfur* were already known as individual remedies, which meant that homeopathic doctors could predict the effect these elements would have together in a compound. In recent years, these predictions have been confirmed in practice, so that *Calcarea sulfurica* has become a significant remedy for children as well as for adults.

Love and Attention

Calcarea children need security in the outside world. They are sensitive about what others think of them, and are generally somewhat

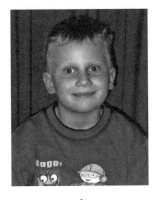

Calc-s.

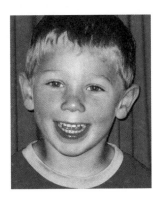

Calc-s.

reserved. *Sulfur* children are mostly open and are concerned with love. They can be loving, but rarely in a selfless way. They themselves remain the focus.

Calcarea sulfurica children show a combination of these characteristics and have, therefore, a great need for love and attention. In this respect, they remind us of *Pulsatilla* children, although the background is different. *Pulsatilla* children are concerned with getting warmth and attention, whereas *Calcarea sulfurica* children are more concerned with their effect on other people. Do you like me? Do you find me good-looking? Am I properly appreciated? These are the questions that *Calcarea sulfurica* children grapple with. The background to all this is judgment and assessment by others and the question of whether they are being taken seriously. So long as they're seen, heard, and loved, they're happy, but when they miss these — even if it's only a subjective feeling — they become unsettled.

Shy, jealous, or aggressive

When *Calcarea sulfurica* children find themselves in a situation in which they have to do without love — either because their parents are unable to give it to them or due to other unfortunate circumstances — they react in different ways. Some withdraw, becoming quiet and shy; some feel excluded and think that other children get more attention than themselves, whereas others become aggressive. Negative attention is also a kind of attention. In their different ways of reacting, these children resemble other remedy types, which fit the reactions described extremely well, such as *Calcarea carbonica*, *Lachesis* or *Lycopodium*. Just like *Lachesis* children, they can complain that they're not being noticed. *Lycopodium* children need power, and behave imperiously due to this feeling, yet they don't actually want to be the "boss." Instead it's a kind of tyranny and awkwardness. The *Sulfur* contribution means that they can think a lot of themselves.

An example of how a *Calcarea sulfurica* picture can arise is when an older child is adopted. As the newcomer to the family, they can get the feeling that the other children — the natural children — are loved more than they are.

Outward appearance is important

Outward appearance plays an important role, even for very young *Calcarea sulfurica* girls. They love pretty clothes, hair decoration, the latest fashion, and so on — the main thing is that they are seen as a beauty. To get attention, they can flirt and ingratiate themselves. Negative remarks about their appearance can damage their self-confidence. In boys, this sensitivity first plays a role in puberty, when they develop an interest in the opposite sex. It's unfortunate that they often suffer from teenage acne, for everyone to see! The good thing about *Calcarea sulfurica* is that it not only helps to restore self-confidence but can also heal the acne. Appearance obviously remains important, but they can handle it better, even if it doesn't match up to their high standards.

Uncertainty about love

Many children are precocious. Who will I marry when I grow up? When is the prince on the white horse coming? *Calcarea sulfurica* children are very vulnerable, especially where a "steady relationship" is involved. Does he love me enough? Will she succumb to the attractions of someone who's better looking than me? At the slightest opportunity for doubt, each child will react in their own way. Some become quiet and withdrawn, whereas others become especially affectionate and try to tie down the other person in any way possible. It all revolves around the same problem: uncertainty about the love of the boyfriend or girlfriend.

Awkward and stubborn

Children often come to see homeopaths because, according to their parents, they "don't feel well in themselves." Difficult behavior is obviously more striking than being quiet and good. At first sight, it's not always clear what's behind the behavior, especially with young children or those with a reserved character. They're awkward and stubborn, and on questioning it turns out that the problems began when another child got more attention than they did. They react by intensifying their demands for confirmation that they're loved and valued. This can go so far that they want to do something to the new brother or sister. They can be particularly obstinate and

restless, and misinterpret every remark. When someone has a different opinion from them, they think this means they're not loved or
valued.

Calcarea sulfurica can help these children to love themselves more
and regain the confidence that they're fine just as they are. This
is the core of the problem. It's difficult for them to really believe
in themselves, and therefore they're dependent on the opinions of
others.

Physical symptoms

Just like *Sulfur* children, they're mostly warm-blooded. Complaints
primarily affect the left side of the body, on the side of the heart,
where the feelings are. They don't tolerate warmth well. They sweat
easily and copiously, especially on exertion. The sweat often smells
strongly. The typical sleeping position is on the back with the arms
above the head, exactly like *Pulsatilla* children. If they're in pain, it's
often of a burning nature. All discharges (for example, with a cold)
are thick, yellow, and in general smell strongly. The skin is the organ
that most frequently shows complaints. We also see here — along
with skin that heals poorly and tends towards inflammation — pustules or acne with yellow fluid and burning pains.

Food and Drink

Calcarea sulfurica children love mostly sweet things and sour fruit
(especially apples) as well as carbohydrate-rich foods. There is
often a dislike of eggs and potatoes.

The Carcinosinum Child

Nosode

"Setting boundaries"

Origin

Carcinosinum is a homeopathic remedy made from tumor cells. Why is this so?

As early as 100 years ago, people were starting to make homeopathic remedies from pathogenic agents. In this way, the homeopathic remedy *Tuberculinum* was created from a culture of tuberculosis and *Medorrhinum* from a culture of gonorrhea. *Tuberculinum* has proved to be a good remedy for the effects of tuberculosis, especially in the descendants (see: *Tuberculinum*), and *Medorrhinum* is good for many typical symptoms resulting from gonorrhea, especially in later generations.

In the same way, research was also undertaken for a remedy that would fit the effects of cancer. This remedy was given the name *Carcinosinum*. Obviously, nosodes are only given as homeopathic preparations that do not contain even a single molecule of the original substance. So *Carcinosinum* no longer contains any tumor cells and works solely on the energetic level!

The various investigations into this remedy have shown that *Carcinosinum* has a very clear remedy picture. We find the complaints and symptoms of this homeopathic remedy in many children (and adults), even when there is no cancer in the family.

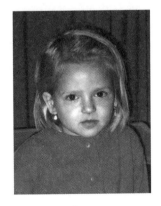

Carc.

Poor sleep

Carcinosinum children are mostly very sweet children who want to fulfill all their parents' wishes. Yet when they're not feeling well, they can be very stubborn. *Carcinosinum* is the most

91

important remedy for babies and children who sleep poorly. When they wake at night, they feel as fit as during the day, so they want to play. Fears can also play a role when they don't want to go to bed. The characteristic sleep position for *Carcinosinum* is with the knees to the chest, exactly the same as for *Medorrhinum* and *Tuberculinum*. A further indication for this remedy is continuous crying in babies. The bigger children love animals, books, and music. When they hear music, they begin to dance, exactly like *Sepia* children. A striking feature is the bluish hue in the sclera (the whites of the eyes), a symptom that often enables us to recognize *Carcinosinum* children the first time we meet them. If they also bite their nails, the decision for this remedy is clear!

Pleasing others

These sensitive children are acutely tuned in to the expectations of their parents or teachers. Therefore, it's very important to teach them to decide for themselves and to stand up for themselves. By nature, they tend to keep their wishes and feelings to themselves and, when necessary, to repress them.

After a dose of this wonderful remedy, we can see how these children blossom. *Carcinosinum* children like to please others since they love peace and harmony and dislike for conflict. Since they have strong intuition and fit in easily, they are in many ways "ideal" children for the people around them. They have a very strong sense of responsibility and are extreme perfectionists. They dislike arriving late and do everything possible to avoid mistakes.

Animals, nature, and music

With their sensitive manner, they're able to empathize not just with people, but also with animals. Indeed, they're usually crazy about animals, although we sometimes find fear of particular animals, such as snakes, mice, and spiders. In general, *Carcinosinum* children are nature lovers. They love storms and thunder and lightning (which can also make them afraid) and feel best by the sea. Most of them love traveling. Music is good for them and they love dancing. Exactly like *Sepia* children, they relax through physical exercise, especially dancing. It's striking that they like reading; they're real bookworms.

Sympathy and worry

Before *Carcinosinum* was discovered, we often mistakenly prescribed *Phosphorus* for this type of child. There are many matching characteristics. Both child types are strongly sympathetic, and can be very worried about their fellow human beings. The fears also show many similarities, such as the fear of serious illness (such as cancer), of bad things happening (such as in frightening movies), of great heights, and of thunderstorms.

Due to their perfectionism and their need to please others, they easily overstep their own boundaries. They leave nothing unfinished in the house and they have difficulty saying no when they're asked to do something. This is their greatest vulnerability: their talent for helping others can easily be abused.

One of the reasons why they're so obedient and eager to help is their lack of self-confidence. They don't dare to be unruly because they think this is no way to behave. This is often connected with their upbringing, since they may have got the feeling that they had to meet the demands made of them at all costs. By nature, they're placid and shy, and would rather give in to pressure than stand up for themselves.

Physical symptoms

Their sensitivity can be expressed in all sorts of allergies, such as hay fever, but also in chronic colds, sinus problems, throat infections, and infections like glandular fever (mononucleosis). It's not just the psychological defense that breaks down, but also the physical defense. They often get the usual childhood illnesses not as children, but later as adults. They overcome infectious illnesses only with great difficulty. They have lots of energy, yet are easily exhausted, so that tiredness is a recurring problem. They tend to get warts, acne, and pustules. Sleep disturbances are common, although it's noticeable that they're completely recovered after a short nap. They often feel good in the evening and can relax well by the sea.

Carcinosinum

Carcinosinum children are liable to develop complications following vaccinations.

Food and Drink

Carcinosinum children have a strong desire for chocolate.

The Causticum Child

Freshly burned lime with bisulfate of potash
(Hahnemann's caustic)

Mineral remedy

"If you hurt someone else, you also hurt me"

Origin

Causticum is one of the discoveries of Samuel Hahnemann. Alongside his occupation as a doctor, he was also a chemist. According to his contemporary, Berzelius, he could have become famous in this field. Using his knowledge of chemistry, he "manufactured" this remedy from natural marble, and it has remained invaluable to this day. Due to its corrosive action, Hahnemann called this substance *Causticum*, which means a caustic or corrosive substance.

Sincerity and sympathy

There are two characteristics that are noticeable even in young *Causticum* children: sincerity and sympathy. They can't lie, even if this would make it easier for them. By nature, they don't mince their words. They always give their opinion, especially concerning sincerity and justice. They're worried by the suffering that they see and feel in the people around them, and they have the feeling that they must do something about it. They can be hard and reserved, yet inside they feel every sorrow.

When they're small and another child starts crying, they cry too, since otherwise they can't stand it. When they're bigger, they try to do something for the other person to soothe their pain. At school, they stand up for weaker children, such as those who are being teased. They feel like Robin Hood.

They do not easily show their own pain and annoyance. Although they have many similarities with *Phosphorus* children, they're less open with their own feelings.

Injustice

As already mentioned, *Causticum* children are sensitive to injustice, both when it directly affects them and when others are the target. They find it easier to stand up for others than for themselves. During puberty, they like starting discussions, not just when they come across injustice, but also because they simply love discussing things. They have fewer fears than *Phosphorus* children. They're sometimes afraid of dogs or the dark. They're not afraid to say what they think, and they don't avoid fights, especially when others are concerned. If there's no way of avoiding it, they'll get involved in a confrontation to — in their eyes — stand up for a just cause.

In puberty *Causticum* children can be a great burden on their parents. They have problems with authority early on, and even as young children they demand an explanation for why they're allowed to do some things and not others. *Causticum* children don't accept authority as such. They experience it as a form of repression and injustice, something they can't tolerate.

Suffering and worry

The problem of suffering and their worry for others can cause them pain. It's not easy for *Causticum* children to let go. They get angry with people who promise the world, but don't keep their promise, and they're annoyed by any kind of hypocrisy they encounter. They get very worried about people close to them. So long as they can express these emotions and can do something to alleviate the pain of the other person, they feel strong. But as soon as they realize that, like Don Quixote, they're fighting windmills, and they realize how powerless they are, their energy can turn inwards against themselves. Stammering occurs in *Causticum* children, frequently due to their agitation or feeling of powerlessness

Learning to set boundaries

Since by nature they feel connected to their fellow human beings, it's difficult for them to set clear boundaries between their own tasks and those of other people. *Causticum* helps them to decide when to invest their energy and when it's better to leave it to someone else. In general, this special remedy can help children to learn about their boundaries. Even though we're all connected with one another, each person has their own task, and we can't simply take over someone else's tasks. Yet obviously we can support others at any time.

Due to excessive worry and because they take on too much, *Causticum* children can get into a state of exhaustion — first, mentally and then also physically. In this phase, many complaints can emerge that are often symbolic of how they feel inside.

Physical symptoms

Causticum children are often recognizable on sight. It's difficult to define the exact features, but we often see an asymmetry of the face and the body. The two sides of the body are different. They often develop skin complaints, such as cracks in the lips, the nostrils, and the anus. But the most characteristic thing is warts on the fingers, right next to the cuticle.

Another weak spot is the muscles. They can suffer from muscle twitches and stammering. These are partially due to agitation, but they're often due to loss of control over the voice muscles. Pains, especially of a drawing and burning kind, can occur in various parts of the body. Restless legs at night in bed are common and are the consequence of feelings such as powerlessness, anger or annoyance, which they can't properly express.

Tiredness is a symptom that gradually increases, first mentally and then also physically. With time, this tiredness can get so bad that they can hardly lift their arms and legs — as if they were paralyzed.

Causticum children generally tend to get hoarse, lose their voice, and become paralyzed, which fortunately clears up on its own in most cases. Facial paralysis after driving with open windows in summer is a notorious *Causticum* symptom. This paralysis, known as Bell's palsy, usually heals on its own. The healing process can be speeded up by *Causticum*, provided that the entire picture fits. A further characteristic localization for paralysis is the bladder. Children can lose urine when they laugh, cough, and so on. *Causticum* can do wonders when given at the right time, and certainly brings relief if it fits the overall picture.

Food and Drink

Causticum children mostly have a desire for smoked food, salt, eggs, cheese, meat, and spicy foods. They don't like sweet things, fish, or vegetables.

The Chamomilla Child

Matricaria recutita, True Chamomile

Plant remedy (Asteraceae family)

"I can't get no satisfaction"

Origin

Chamomile belongs to the Compositae family (Asteraceae), a large plant family that is widespread nearly worldwide. The Compositae family is also known as the aster, daisy, or sunflower family. Many members of the Compositae family are typical child remedies, which means that they're often required in childhood, and they fit the typical problems that children have.

It's most likely that true chamomile was originally found only in south and south-east Europe but as the healing effects of the plant became known, it gained in popularity all over the world. Nowadays, this plant is cultivated worldwide, except at the poles and in the tropics. The medicinal components of chamomile have anti-inflammatory, anti-bacterial, and antispasmodic effects.

The active ingredients in the plant — for example, as chamomile tea — and also the homeopathic remedy (mostly in the potencies 6x and 12x) are often used for children suffering from toothache, stomach cramps, and ear infections. If the child also shows the typical behavior described below, *Chamomilla* is the remedy of choice. *Chamomilla* is, however, often prescribed in error, particularly when children are behaving quite differently than we would expect from the remedy picture. It's very unlikely that such children could profit from *Chamomilla*, since in these cases another homeopathic remedy would be more suitable.

True *Chamomilla* children are those who show *Chamomilla* behavior not just when ill, but who in all respects correspond to the *Chamomilla* type.

Strong and independent

Chamomilla children want to be strong and independent, which they basically are anyway. This issue is found in all plants from the Compositae family. The children are afraid of being weak, especially physically. Physical changes or pain are, therefore, experienced as a terrible threat. They get the feeling that their whole world, their security, is being attacked.

Complaints occur mainly when the pattern of their lives changes. Teething is normally a difficult time, as is each of the subsequent developmental steps.

Their reaction is expressed as protest! Nobody suffers more than they do, nothing can help. Every possible means of expressing rage is used: screaming, hitting, biting, and scratching. The only possibility of calming them down is to pick them up, move around, and rock them a little.

Miracle cure

If there is one remedy that can convince doctors and parents of the healing effect of homeopathy, that remedy is *Chamomilla*. Imagine that a child showing the symptoms described above is given a globule of *Chamomilla* 30c or several doses of 6x or 12x: anyone witnessing the effects will think that the child has been given a tranquilizer. The remarkable thing is that these children can then proceed without problem to the next stage of development and will behave according to their age. Obviously, the remedy should be repeated as soon as the healing process grinds to a halt.

Challenging

One of the problems that we often encounter in children who need a remedy from the Composite family (Asteraceae) is that they have problems setting boundaries. Either they haven't learned how to do this or they don't feel strong enough. They quickly interpret things as threats and then seek protection from other people, even when these people then overstep the child's boundaries. This behavior of overstepping the boundaries doesn't apply to *Chamomilla* children at all. They want to forestall the other person and so attempt to defend themselves by challenging and preemptively going on the attack. This is not to dominate the other person but to show themselves that they are strong enough and are, therefore, not in danger. The aim of the attack and the challenge is not a real fight — it's just a game. It's a bit like a boxer who needs a sparring partner to prepare for the real thing.

Difficult to satisfy

Due to their character, *Chamomilla* children are difficult to satisfy. Most children have some activity, such as a sport or a hobby, where they find some peace and contentment. *Chamomilla* children, however, simply can't find satisfaction in anything — they're continually getting into conflicts. It's a fight against inner disquiet, a search for relief from the pain that they so easily experience. Their nervous system is oversensitive and they feel every hurt more intensely than other children. The Rolling Stones' song "I can't get no satisfaction" perfectly sums up their predicament.

They resist their own development. All Asteraceae children have this problem. They really just want to remain children, without responsibility. They need other people to take the blame for their suffering. Not for nothing is *Chamomilla* the most important remedy for teething and for every developmental step.

Physical symptoms

As already mentioned, every phase of growth or rather every developmental step is associated with pain for *Chamomilla* children. Every change brings with it complaints, even natural functions such as urination, defecation, and menstruation. Complaints during teething (often accompanied by diarrhea), indigestion, and complaints during urination and defecation are characteristic for *Chamomilla*. They express their pain noisily and rudely. But it's best not to try and console them, never mind looking at them, because they think this invites dependence. And this is exactly what they don't want! The pain, moreover, gives them a reason to complain.

Chamomilla infants clench their fists, stiffen themselves and arch backwards. The older children can't sit still — instead, they run around and want most of all to be carried (but not consoled!). They can be extremely loud and their screaming goes right through you. Absolutely nothing can calm the child (except *Chamomilla*), yet they demand instant relief!

When the teeth have come through and the body is freed from the struggle, they feel relieved. They feel better for physical activity.

Another clinical picture for which *Chamomilla* can bring rapid relief is middle-ear infection, always assuming that the behavior matches that described above!

Food and Drink

Chamomilla children desire cold and sour drinks. Besides this, they like bread and have a dislike of soup and meat.

Teething

If there is one thing for which many parents use homeopathy to treat their children, it's problems during teething. *Chamomilla* is for many parents a magic word. When they've experienced how quickly a weepy, whining, and often troublesome child calms down again after a dose of *Chamomilla*, they really know how well homeopathy can work.

Apparently the British royal family once employed a homeopathic doctor for this reason. A young prince around 1850 was apparently a troublesome *Chamomilla* child who was impossible to deal with. The doctors were powerless, yet a nurse knew what to do: *Chamomilla*!

Chamomilla is unfortunately not always the best remedy for teething problems. If *Chamomilla* doesn't help, please see a professional homeopath in your neighborhood.

The Cina Child

Artemisia cina, Levant wormseed

Plant remedy (Asteraceae Family)

"Contra"

Origin

Doctors used to obtain this plant from the eastern Mediterranean. Although it could be found in European countries, the best quality came from the "Levant." Warm air does this plant good, which also applies to children needing this remedy.

Its English name is "wormseed." People have used it since time immemorial to combat intestinal parasites such as worms. Linnaeus called it *Artemisia contra*, an abbreviation for "*Artemisia contra vermes*" ("Artemisia against worms"). And indeed an indication for the homeopathic remedy *Cina* is the susceptibility to intestinal parasites.

The word "contra" fits this type of child perfectly. *Chamomilla* is well known as a remedy that is helpful for children who are troublesome when ill. Yet *Cina* children can be a whole lot more troublesome than *Chamomilla* children. Both *Chamomilla* and *Cina* belong to the Compositae family, the members of which have much in common. They are typical child remedies that are frequently needed when children become aware of their place and their relationship to those around them. They have already built up their own "I," and now have the feeling that they need to protect themselves against the outside world. Children from the Compositae family do this with their immune system, both literally and figuratively. Defense is a natural reaction to threatening situations. Every change and every new environment is for them primarily a potential threat.

Touchy: oversensitive, irritated, prickly

Cina children are very sensitive to their environment, both on a physical and emotional level. Just like *Chamomilla* children, they have a very delicate nervous system. The difference between the

103

two types is in the intensity of the reaction and the type of physical complaints. As long as they're healthy and are in a calm, harmonious environment, they are contented. Then they're easy-going and friendly, since they're not particularly annoying by nature.

They have a strong desire for safety and security. It's only when something of this is destroyed that the other side of their character comes out. We could say that they resist the independence developing within them. *Cina* children like to hold others — preferably their parents — responsible for their welfare and well-being. If they're not feeling well, that's someone else's fault. The first sign is that they don't want to be touched. Especially combing or brushing their hair is an imposition; they scream at the top of their voice and do everything to prevent it. Pain, such as during teething, is something they tolerate poorly. It's noticeable that they often pick their nose.

Nasty and stubborn

If a problem can't be solved, the child reacts with increasing vehemence. Not just touch, but also eye contact arouses intense resistance and can lead to loud shrieking, initially only with strangers, later also with acquaintances and in the family. Everything is taken negatively, even well-meaning cuddles! *Cina* children are real troublemakers. They ask for something only to throw it away as soon as they get it, even if it's their favorite toy! *Chamomilla* children also throw things around, but *Cina* children can even aim at other peo-

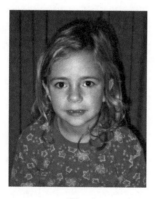

Cina

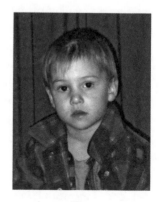

Cina

ple. Their reaction is so nasty and extreme that they try and hit someone. Absolutely nothing you do is right for them. They scream, throw, bite — they show their discontent in every imaginable way, as if someone was challenging or terrorizing them. They even cry or grind their teeth at night in their sleep. In this way, they demonstrate their dissatisfaction even when at rest.

Cina children are possibly the most annoying type of child when they're not feeling well. But it's marvelous to see how they come round after taking *Cina*. This remedy helps them to become more independent, and to take on more responsibility for their own life. They're basically very lively children with a strong will and temperament!

Physical symptoms

The most striking physical complaints are the oversensitivity to touch, especially on the head, and the tendency to worm infections. These infections are often accompanied by an itchy nose and an overpowering urge to pick the nose. They also complain frequently of stomach ache and have a soft stool. They get dark rings round the eyes, and the skin round the nose and mouth appears blue-white. This together with their behavior enables homeopathic doctors to recognize this type of child.

Exactly like *Chamomilla* children, they often have complaints from teething. They can go completely stiff with rage, and we can also see tense muscles when they cough or when they're being looked at. Another typical symptom is frequent yawning when they aren't feeling well.

Serious neurological complaints can also fit this remedy, especially symptoms of epilepsy. Children with this illness suddenly wake at night as if frightened by something and then they scream; after sitting up, they become stiff and rigid.

At night, they can rage and scream, even making noises in their sleep. Grinding of the teeth occurs with *Cina*, as well as also with some other remedy pictures, such as *Belladonna* (an equally intense remedy) and *Tuberculinum*. Warmth, movement, and lying on the stomach all bring them some relief.

Food and Drink

It's striking that newborn *Cina* children refuse the breast. In general, they tolerate milk poorly.

Older children can have an enormous appetite, although they hardly gain weight. There can be a noticeable desire for salt.

The Cuprum Child

Copper (Cu). Mineral remedy

"Rules and Rituals"

Origin

Copper was one of the first metals to be used by mankind. The name comes from Cyprus, the island where long ago large amounts of copper were discovered. In nature, it occurs not only in the pure form but also bound as minerals (such as chalcopyrite, chalcosite, cuprite, malachite and azurite). It is a soft, elastic, and malleable metal, which is, after silver, the best conductor of heat and electricity. From time immemorial, copper has been used for basic commodities such as bowls and vases. Nowadays copper is used in gas, water, and heating pipes, as well as for electrical installations. The special thing about copper is its corrosion resistance. This comes from its ability to build a stable surface layer that protects the metal from further corrosion. This protective quality of copper is reflected in the remedy picture.

Strong but sensitive to change

Cuprum children are by nature strong-willed and generally have a positive character. They like to joke yet their anger is also hard for

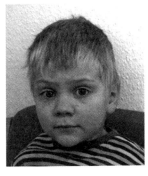
Cupr-br.

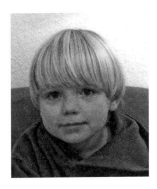
Cupr-c.

them to hide. They have fixed ideas and find it easiest when things run according to plan. Then they know where they are, and they can't be taken by surprise. They love security, exactly like *Calcarea carbonica* children, but they are even more inclined to look to rules and rituals for support. Their reaction to change is also stronger than for *Calcarea carbonica* children. In this, they're similar to *Chamomilla* and *Belladonna* children. Attack is the best form of defense. Yelling, biting, spitting — anything goes when they're furious.

It's not surprising that *Cuprum* — along with *Chamomilla*, *Nux vomica*, and *Belladonna* — is one of the most important remedies for infants with colic.

Routine and rules

The desire for routines and rules is obvious at all times. They don't like it when things don't go according to plan. They'll always try, no matter how young they are, to meet the demands made of them. At school, for example, they do everything to get their work done. They need recognition and can't tolerate criticism. They follow the rules set by the teacher. When other children break the rules, they don't hesitate to point this out to them. As far as the teachers are concerned, they are the ideal pupils — if the teacher needs someone to supervise the class, these children can be relied on.

Spasmodic

In their tendency toward perfectionism and their need for recognition, *Cuprum* children like to have things under control, including their emotions. They quickly become worried about everything they still have to do, which can lead to fear of the future, of accidents, illness, and death. Their original liveliness then disappears and turns into a more serious attitude.

If too much is expected of them, they desperately do their best to meet the demands. Physically, this can be expressed in various complaints — cramps, nail-biting, stammering, stuttering, muscle twitches, asthma, and also epilepsy. When the fury is suppressed, it can come out as paroxysmal holding of the breath. This goes so far that the child becomes blue and even unconscious. So much nervous energy lies behind the anger and they need to get rid of it!

Cuprum children quickly become nasty, and easily feel attacked or criticized.

Generally, it's best not to ask too much of our children, especially when they're *Cuprum* children who don't know how to deal with it at all.

Smoothing troubled waters

When there are tensions in the family or at school, they quickly feel responsible and do their best to calm things down, even if it means they themselves have to walk on eggshells.

Cuprum children are quite self-confident and like to take control of things. They can, therefore, be reasonably dominant. The tone in which they put their questions can sometimes seem like a command rather than a question. Everything has to do with their wish for independence and control. It's difficult for them to trust others completely. On the one hand, they tend to be reserved and don't like to be touched by strangers; but on the other hand, they can often resolve a tense situation with a well-chosen joke. With their behavior, they try to keep their feelings, which can be very strong, under control.

Physical symptoms

All complaints are associated with cramps. First, the muscles are affected — calf cramps, neck pain, headaches, and so on — then later also the deeper parts of the body.

Tension in the chest can lead to asthma or even cardiovascular disease. Since their blood vessels get cramped easily, *Cuprum* children often have, for example, (icy) cold hands and feet. At the peak of the cramps, epileptic fits are possible.

Cuprum children feel better from physical exercise, massage, gentle touch, and showering. This helps them reduce the tension they feel.

Food and Drink

They prefer cold drinks, cold food, sweet things, and meat. They don't much like warm or cooked food. Cold drinks relieve various complaints such as coughing, nausea, and spasms.

The Ferrum metallicum Child

Iron (Fe). Mineral remedy

"Fighter by nature"

Origin

Iron occurs everywhere on earth, as an ore as well as in all living organisms. It's the fourth most common element on the planet. In the human body, iron is especially important for the red blood cells. Iron helps the blood to transport oxygen to the tissues. The red color of our blood comes from the iron! That's why children with anemia look so pale — due to the lack of iron.

Since the start of the Iron Age, this metal has been used to manufacture tools and weapons. Therefore, the same substance is used on the one hand to construct things — iron in the form of steel accounts for the stability of many constructions — and on the other hand, in the form of weapons, to destroy things. Iron represents the male power to act and create things. We can find many hints in our language about the *Ferrum* type. Think of "pumping iron," "Iron Lady" (Margaret Thatcher), or children with a "will of iron."

Will of iron

Ferrum children not only have a will of iron, they also know exactly what they want to achieve when they act. They're particularly goal-oriented. When they get something into their head, they'll do everything to reach their goal, just like *Nux vomica* children. This is an enormous force, and it's not always easy for parents to get along with their *Ferrum* children. They require clarity and boundaries. It's not that these children deliberately try to overstep the boundaries or to offend somebody. They simply have their eyes fixed on a goal of their own and want to achieve this. They are, however, less complicated than *Nux vomica* and *Chamomilla* children, since there is no complicated emotional pattern behind their behavior. They're just single-minded, that's all! Whether it's a small child trying to grab the dice or a teenager keen to finish his homework, they stick at it until they're through!

110

Competent

Ferrum children are "competent," by which I mean they're brave, determined, and steadfast. When they want something, they fight their way through any obstacle. This is their strength as well as their weakness. There is a lot of strength in these children, but with their compulsion to perform and their staying power, they run the risk of going beyond their limits.

They think that problems always have a solution and they look particularly for practical solutions. It's obviously important for their development that they learn to fit in, which costs their parents extra energy and attention. They need to learn to judge the benefit and appropriateness of what is being asked of them. Despite their drive, they have considerable trouble achieving the goals in life that they've set themselves.

Difficult task

Ferrum children are looking for a challenge. They are fighters in the literal as well as the figurative sense. With their perfectionism and their stamina, they're always setting themselves tasks in which something is expected of them. This applies to the physical as well as the intellectual level. They carry out their work with much discipline, and they stay on top of things. *Ferrum* children are good organizers and they prefer clear structures.

Opposition and criticism

Since *Ferrum* children work hard and like to have a goal to work towards, they experience any opposition as criticism. This annoys them greatly. They tolerate opposition poorly and everything that might restrict them — sometimes even the slightest noise (such as the rustling of a newspaper) — disturbs them. When they get nasty, their entire energy is channeled into aggression, which they express in words and possibly also in deeds. Therefore, they like to be alone when they're not feeling well. They tend to interpret negative remarks, especially criticism, in a very personal way. The thought that they might not be good is unbearable for *Ferrum* children.

111

By hook or by crook

We find their weaknesses where their strengths are. For *Ferrum* children, it's the way they like to complete their tasks. They're rarely pleased with what they've done. Tasks must always be finished off. We find a similar sense of duty in *Kalium carbonicum* children, but there it's not such a "must." *Ferrum* people feel they have to solve the problem otherwise they can't stop — in any case, they won't allow themselves to stop. The danger lies in the fact that they're always forcing themselves to go beyond their limits. They don't want to make any mistakes, especially not when they're being put to the test, as in an examination. Yet due to their compulsion, they overshoot the mark.

Physical symptoms

Ferrum children easily get problems to do with the blood, such as anemia, nosebleed, and bleeding in general. It's striking that they have red cheeks that feel cold instead of warm. The circulation is very sensitive, so that they often have congestion and pulsations in various parts of the body. When *Ferrum* children have gone beyond their limits, they can become extremely tired, cold, and weak. Normally, their complaints worsen with the slightest physical exertion, yet they can also get pains that force them to take some exercise. They generally feel at their best when they're moving around slowly. Since they often suffer from sensitivity to foods, it's always worth thinking of *Ferrum* for food allergies. They can also get complaints like nausea and diarrhea.

Food and Drink

Ferrum children love tomatoes and sour food. They mostly don't want eggs, which they tolerate poorly, and the same applies to fat.

The Graphites Child

Graphite, Carbon (C). Mineral remedy

"The foundation of the sense of self-esteem"

Origin

Carbon is the foundation of all living organisms and is one of the key elements in biochemistry, the study of the chemical processes in living things. Carbon compounds in both living and non-living things are so important they have their own separate branch of chemistry called organic chemistry. Carbon has special characteristics and forms the stable framework of the human body.

In nature, the pure element carbon occurs in several forms. The two best known are: graphite, a black, soft
material from which pencils are made; and diamond, the hardest-known mineral, which is also as transparent as glass. A better comparison of the soft and the hard sides of *Graphites* is probably with the softest and hardest pencil.

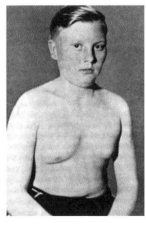

Graph.

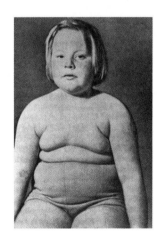

Graph.

113

Self-Esteem

The homeopathic remedy *Graphites* is closely associated with the self-esteem of a child. A child with problems of self-esteem might need *Graphites* or another carbon compound. It's therefore closely related to *Calcarea carbonica* and *Barium carbonicum*. In practice, it's not always easy for the doctor to make a clear distinction between these remedies.

Graphites fits the stage of life when the child develops a sense of identity, some time in the sixth or seventh year of life. If the child gets the right support and motivation, in this case especially from the father figure, it will develop well. Unfortunately, this is not always the case. The absence of the father — literally or figuratively — or exaggerated support from him can cause an imbalance. This means that two types of child can develop, both of which need *Graphites* to restore balance.

Let's begin with the stable type, who shouldn't need any (more) of the remedy.

Stable and self-confident

The key issue with *Graphites* children is self-confidence, the feeling that they think themselves "good." When they're balanced, their self-confidence is fine. They're free of doubts and they trust themselves. What they do and who they are is "good." These children have strong opinions of their own and can be very stubborn. Not because they're obstinate or rebellious, but simply because they think that their opinion is the right one. These *Graphites* children can be astonishingly ambitious.

That they're so worldly-wise doesn't mean that they're not sensitive. Other people's troubles can affect them deeply and good music can move them to tears. They are pleasant, sociable children.

Graphites children can work hard; they work slowly, but at the same time tenaciously and persistently. They prefer practical activities most of all and can be very precise, almost fussy. They like to do something useful. They're real doers.

The two descriptions below of unsettled *Graphites* children mostly occur in different children, but can also occur in the same child, depending on mood and circumstances.

Soft and oversensitive

If *Graphites* children receive too little support and motivation — the critical stage is the sixth or seventh year — they can develop in two directions: they either become soft and oversensitive or hard and unfeeling.

The oversensitive *Graphites* children resemble *Pulsatilla* children. They're shy and cry easily, sometimes at the slightest provocation. Hearing or seeing something bad, such as a depressing film or a sad story, can unsettle them. But they completely lose their self-control when their self-worth is under attack, such as when they're being criticized or reprimanded.

If they're asked why they're crying, they often don't know themselves. They can give vent to their emotions by speaking about it with a parent or someone they trust. They need to communicate with somebody; otherwise they tend to repress their feelings. They enjoy being caressed. In this phase, their desire to work is hardly noticeable, and they would really rather do nothing at all.

In contrast to *Pulsatilla* children, the problems with *Graphites* children are closely connected to their self-esteem, whereas *Pulsatilla* children tend to be looking for love and attention.

Hard and rigid

The other extreme can be seen in those *Graphites* children who were brought up harshly or who have learned to harden themselves as a reaction to traumatic experiences.

When brought up harshly, the children rigidly hang on to the rules and norms that they picked up at home, without thinking whether they themselves really support them. They follow in the footsteps of their father or mother and adopt their point of view. It's difficult for them to adapt to new situations. Their reaction is then to "grit their teeth and get on with it." They protect themselves by letting nothing get to them and clinging to what they believe is good and right. Their stubbornness can get so bad that even punishment no longer has any effect. They even laugh about it! At such times, they're absolutely not interested in consolation or contact.

The meaning of life

In the phase around the sixth or seventh year of life, the father stands symbolically for "God." He's the highest authority for the child. We can often see in *Graphites* children a religious sensibility. Even as young children, they're inquisitive about the meaning of life and they search for a deeper meaning. From the moment when they perceive their father as authority, they realize that there are other authorities such as the teacher, the priest, or God. *Graphites* children are very sensitive, although they don't show it. They react sensitively to criticism and they always need extra encouragement.

When children in this phase become unsettled, and self-esteem is the origin of the problems, *Graphites* helps them to become the stable person that they basically are.

Physical symptoms

Graphites is known especially for its curative action on skin diseases. These occur in children mostly on the head. Skin diseases such as cradle cap, milk crust, seborrheic eczema, seborrheic dermatitis, and atopic eczema (neurodermatitis, atopic dermatitis, and endogenous eczema) occur frequently in *Graphites* children. The cracks in the skin are characteristic and can appear anywhere, especially behind the ears and the anus. Rashes often exude a yellow, sticky fluid. The nails of the hands and feet are sometimes thick, yellow, and crumbly. Ear infections are frequently accompanied by a discharge from the ear and can persist for a long time. The left ear is particularly sensitive. The tonsils tend to be somewhat swollen.

Graphites children are by nature rather heavily built and tend to become overweight when not feeling well. They're somewhat slower than average in both mental and physical functioning. Although they love physical activity, excessive effort or too much exercise has an adverse effect on them because they have a tendency to complaints of the bones.

If the remedy is indicated, it can not only completely heal the skin and other physical complaints, but also leave the child beaming with self-confidence!

Food and Drink

They mostly have a preference for sweet things — or sometimes it's the exact opposite. They have a desire for "simple" food, chicken, and hot milk. They don't like meat and fish. There can also be a dislike of warm food and salty food.

The Helium Child

Helium (He). Noble Gas. Mineral remedy

"Living completely in their own world"

Origin

Helium is an inert gas that was first discovered in 1868 in the spectral line of the sun. The name comes from the Greek: *"helios"* means "sun" or "sun-god."

According to modern astronomical knowledge, helium was created in the sun by the fusion of hydrogen atoms. The energy released in this reaction is the energy of the sun. This process occurs not just in the sun but in all the stars in the universe and it converts hydrogen, the smallest and most common element in the universe, into the second element, helium. This is the first step in the formation of the bigger and heavier elements familiar to us from the periodic table.

Exactly like all other noble gases — neon, argon, krypton, xenon, and radon — helium is a colorless and odorless gas. Due to its low weight and incombustibility, it's used to fill balloons. Hydrogen is lighter but also more inflammable, as is well known from the catastrophe when the Zeppelin exploded.

In liquid form — under 4 degrees Kelvin — helium develops striking properties. It loses its electrical resistance and becomes a superconductor, creeping up the walls of capillary tubes as if challenging gravity. An amusing anecdote is the story of a child who reacted well to *Helium*. One of the symptoms leading to the choice of the correct remedy was that the child crept over the earth, closely following the unevenness of the ground, including vertically, just like liquid helium.

No connections

One of the properties of this inert gas is that it doesn't form compounds with other elements. It is, as it were, self-contained. This

comes from the fact that because its electron shell is already complete, it does not react with other elements..

We find these characteristics in the picture of children who need
Helium as a homeopathic remedy. They feel happy in their own
world, just like an unborn child in the womb. They drift around in
the warm amniotic fluid, knowing that they're cared for and nour-
ished. This picture can easily arise in people who don't seriously
want to tackle life on earth. They're no longer floating, but they
don't want to be confronted with the tough reality of life on earth.
Helium children choose their own world, a world that they know
from the time when they were not yet born. It may be that by nature
they don't have the strength to accept the world as it is, or that
they had distressing experiences as very young children. In the latter
case, it's a matter of fleeing from a threatening situation.

Autism

It's very difficult for other people to establish contact with them.
One of the illnesses that can occur with *Helium* is autism, a psychological condition in which someone cannot be reached by others
and, superficially, doesn't show any need for communication.

This picture can have various causes. Children with a congenital
or acquired mental disability can fit the *Helium* picture as well as
children who, after taking medical drugs, have fallen into a state of
semi-consciousness. A patient who had become completely withdrawn after receiving a certain medication later regained conscious-
ness after taking a dose of *Helium* in homeopathic form.

A further possible cause for the *Helium* picture is a long period of
isolation from normal life, such as in children who have spent a
long time in hospital or in prison.

We can see from the examples above that *Helium* is not a remedy for
self-treatment. Besides, there are other homeopathic remedies that
might also be appropriate. Only someone with sound knowledge
of homeopathic remedies can make an informed choice between
the various remedies based on a correct assessment of the clinical
picture.

Physical symptoms

There are only a few physical symptoms known for *Helium*. The emotional picture is strongly predominant. Several symptoms that make us think of *Helium* are: feeling of lightness, sensation of floating, and the need to make contact with the earth, as described above in the case of the child who crept like a snake over the ground. A noticeably high-pitched voice, like Donald Duck, also fits *Helium*. When people inhale helium gas, they automatically get this kind of voice.

The Hydrogenium Child

Hydrogen (H). Mineral remedy

"Not yet down here on earth"

Origin

Hydrogen (H) is the smallest atom. It doesn't occur in a free form on earth, whereas the sun and stars are composed mainly of hydrogen. Hydrogen turns into helium by nuclear fusion. As an elemental gas (H_2), it's so light that it's the only element able to escape the earth's gravitational field. Together with oxygen, hydrogen forms a special substance: water (H_2O), which is the source of all life on earth and without which life would not be possible.

According to current theories about the origin of life in the universe, hydrogen is in actual fact the first element. The other elements were gradually formed by nuclear fusion.

Here we can't help comparing the creation of human beings. Our body with all its different cells originated in the beginning from a single fertilized egg cell.

Conception and birth

At conception, the sperm cell and the egg cell fuse together. The single cell that then emerges contains all the characteristics of the future human being. Just as the hydrogen atom feels itself connected to the universe, so do human beings still feel themselves during the act of creation to be part of the whole.

Hydrogenium seems to be a remedy that is suitable for problems during conception and birth. Problems to do with conception can lead to the child not properly arriving on earth, as if they're floating: "Actually, I'm still on another planet."

Older children, who don't feel grounded on earth, can also "float" when they use certain drugs. They can have the feeling that their soul is separated from their body.

121

Dreaming and escaping

Unity with the whole can be experienced as a feeling of ecstasy. In the final analysis, every human being has an inner need to return to this condition of unity. All religions (religion means reconnection) aim to merge with the whole, with God. Yet when this condition arises from not wanting to be on earth, it can easily lead to a loss of the sense of reality.

These children begin to dream. They have problems coping with everyday life, and they search with might and main for ways of escaping the harsh reality. In this state, they can develop the feeling of being connected with everything and everyone. They appear to be able to read other people's thoughts – which is sometimes actually true! – and to be able to move effortlessly through space and time. This can produce a marvelous feeling of freedom and connectedness.

Isolation

The flight from earthly things can also lead to the child isolating itself. The need for unity, which is very strong in *Hydrogenium* children, makes the separation particularly noticeable. Life on earth is full of contrasts and conflicts. Various fears can arise, especially of loneliness and of being abandoned. The feeling of body and soul being separated increases the isolation even more. A constant, restless search is the result, in which the child seeks various forms of unity and connection so as to suppress these fears.

Hydrogenium can help children suffering in this way to establish a better connection to their earthly body. This grounding once again puts them in a position to accept life as it is and to face up to conflicts.

Physical symptoms

In general, *Hydrogenium* children feel better in the open air, although they can't tolerate cold and frost well. They find heavy cloud and strong sun unpleasant, and they're very sensitive to the weather.

Physical exertion such as climbing stairs, light, clothing, and touch can worsen the condition of *Hydrogenium* children, whereas they feel better when they lie down quietly. The complaints occur suddenly

122

and then disappear. It's mainly the right half of the body that's affected. Apart from sleeplessness and — in older girls — problems with the periods, there are only a few physical symptoms known for this remedy.

Food and Drink

Hydrogenium children often have a strong desire for pineapple and cold drinks. In older children, there can be a desire for hashish. They have an aversion to spicy food, warm food, and drink.

They have a love-hate relationship to sour food and they can also get complaints from it.

The Hyoscyamus niger Child

Black henbane. Plant remedy (Solanaceae family)

"Wants to be loved at all costs"

Origin

Black henbane (*Hyoscyamus*), thorn apple or jimsonweed (*Stramonium*), as well as deadly nightshade (*Belladonna*), are the best-known members of the nightshade family used as remedies in homeopathy. In the past, these plants were known as, for example, devil's thorn and devil's snare, and in Germany were used in "witches' brew," where their psychoactive nature was exploited. Nowadays, they're still used as drugs, although this is strictly not recommended due to the high concentration of toxins in them. They're obviously much stronger than the edible vegetable nightshade plants, such as potatoes, eggplant, tomatoes, and red pepper.

As remedies, members of the nightshade family can help children — and also adults — to restore the balance between the dark and light sides of their nature. In the picture of *Hyoscyamus*, we can see many animal elements, especially from snakes. The similarity between *Hyoscyamus* and *Lachesis* (bushmaster snake) is so great that it's difficult to tell them apart.

Black henbane has a moody nature, which can be seen clearly on fallow land: first it appears in large numbers but the next moment it's completely disappeared! In the remedy picture of this plant, we can see something of its moody ways. One of the alkaloids, hyoscyamine, is also used as an analgesic and anesthetic. In the past, it was used to make remedies for tooth-ache and rheumatism.

Energetic kids who are "all there"

Hyoscyamus children are lively kids. They're bursting with energy and they really want to be seen and heard by the people around them. They're certainly "all there." Embarrassment and shyness are unknown to them. As soon as they can speak, they're telling anyone who will listen what's on their mind, just like *Lachesis* children. They're spontaneous and devoid of timidity.

When they know a song, they'll sing joyfully to anyone, or similarly they'll demonstrate some new dance steps that they've just learned. They like being the center of attention. In their openness and directness they're very similar to *Phosphorus* children, although they're maybe less sensitive to the suffering of others. They observe the world in a bright-eyed, unselfconscious and naïve way.

ATTENTION!

The demand for attention from *Hyoscyamus* children is considerable. Basically, they can't live without attention. These children are charming and cute; they know how to score by getting laughs. They're often born clowns and entertainers. But as with every important character trait, this is also their weakness. When they aren't getting the required attention on their own account, they'll do everything in their power to get it. Being seen is for them the same as being loved. They can't imagine that other people could love them if these people are not looking at them and listening to them. We find this issue in an almost identical form in *Lachesis* (and to a lesser extent in other snake remedies). The essential difference is that *Lachesis* children want to play the boss in their own circle. *Hyoscyamus* children don't have their own patch — in principle, they feel at home with the people who love them.

Feeling neglected

These children need the remedy *Hyoscyamus* when they're feeling neglected. This is often the case after the birth of a little brother or sister, but it can also result from a break-up. When one of the parents leaves, *Hyoscyamus* children can interpret this to mean they're no longer loved. They become quiet and unapproachable, yet they can still have violent fits of jealousy or destructiveness.

To get attention, they play the clown or the buffoon, or they act up. "Any kind of attention is better than none at all!" Small children crawl around everywhere, over the furniture and even over people. When *Hyoscyamus* children haven't learned how to establish contact with people in a friendly way, they can attempt to impose themselves shamelessly. They do this by offensive language, singing obscene songs, or even — when the children are a bit older — by

125

provocative clothing. They're not so much interested in the sexual aspect but rather they want attention.

Destructive

When they don't succeed in this way, the children can become very bad, especially with their parents and people who they are close to and from whom they expect to be loved. They throw a tantrum and use crude language. They can also take it out on somebody by hurting them or smashing things.

When *Hyoscyamus* children retreat into themselves, there's often no way of telling what's going on inside. They just sit quietly and stare. Many children seem to be preoccupied by something. One child might be completely fixated on their finger, another is always counting things. One characteristic symptom that indicates *Hyoscyamus* is tugging, for example, a blanket or pullover, or grasping imaginary things in the air. At night, their feelings erupt in the form of laughing, shouting, grinding their teeth, and so on. Of course, it's very important that these children get the appropriate professional help in good time, otherwise their fantasy world can get out of control and they can no longer be reached. The homeopathic remedy *Hyoscyamus* can certainly play a supporting role here.

Rejection

The problem with *Hyoscyamus* children is that they quickly feel rejected. By nature, they have difficulties loving themselves, and they seek reassurance in the outside world. If someone else gets more attention than they do, this is a sign for them that they aren't loved or that they're being let down. At the slightest opportunity, they think a friendship is over or that the other person wants to offend them. A rejection in affairs of the heart can really drive them crazy, and can lead to aggressiveness against the other person or themselves. Jealousy and mistrust are easily aroused in them and their reactions are moody, just as their emotional life can be so intense and changeable.

As soon as the remedy picture is clear — and the parents' help is decisive here — balance can be restored. At the bottom of their heart, *Hyoscyamus* children don't really want to hurt other people, they're simply looking for love and attention.

Physical symptoms

Hyoscyamus has a big influence on the nervous system, as is already known from herbal medicine. Complaints to do with muscle cramps or involuntary movements fit this picture. An example of oversensitivity might be the inability to tolerate the scent of flowers, which can make Hyoscyamus children giddy. Epilepsy is another illness of the nervous system that can be treated with Hyoscyamus, as long as the remedy is indicated for that particular child.

Another physical complaint is dry, convulsive coughing, often associated with nervousness, which can lead to a sense of constriction. Lying down makes it worse, whereas sitting up improves it noticeably.

If Hyoscyamus children don't have an outlet for their feelings, this can lead to sleep disturbances, since they're unable to calm down. Emotional upset can even cause inflammation.

If the nervous system breaks down, the bladder and gut can be "paralyzed" for a time, such that the child cannot hold its urine and feces.

Food and Drink

The aversion to water is a strong indication for Hyoscyamus! This is an uncommon symptom and any homeopathic doctor seeing it will immediately think of Hyoscyamus.

Spicy foods should be avoided because Hyoscyamus children don't react well to them.

The Ignatia Child

Ignatia amara, St. Ignatius bean. Plant remedy (Loganiaceae family)

"Sensitive and idealistic"

Origin

Ignatia belongs to the Loganiaceae family, like *Nux vomica* and *Gelsemium*. These three plants all contain strychnine. This substance explains the cramps that we see with this remedy. In terms of its effect, *Ignatia* comes between the other two remedies. In terms of intensity, *Ignatia* is stronger than *Gelsemium*, but not as explosive as *Nux vomica*. It's like a repressed intensity that — depending on the situation — can either turn inwards or erupt outwards in moody outbursts. The common themes of the Loganiaceae are competition and perfectionism.

Ignatia is obtained from the pulverized seeds of the Ignatius bean tree, which grows in the Philippines and is named after Ignatius of Loyola, the founder of the order of the Jesuits.

Striving for lofty goals

Ignatia children want to reach the goals that they've set themselves. They have a particular, idealized picture of "how things should be," which they do their best to achieve. With great sensitivity, they apprehend what's expected of them and how other people are feeling. By nature, they like doing good, and they're affected by the suffering of others. They're less persistent than *Nux vomica* children and gentler. Yet they're not as docile as *Pulsatilla* and *Carcinosinum* children. They can certainly be intense and extremely industrious. If there's a competition, they want to win.

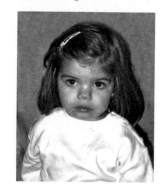

Ign.

They're idealistic children who wholeheartedly support, for example, projects to combat animal abuse. They go to extremes to accomplish these goals and are extremely disappointed if something goes wrong. They really take it to heart.

Sensitive to criticism

There are few children who are as sensitive to criticism as *Ignatia* children. *Staphisagria* children and *Carcinosinum* children are also very sensitive in this respect, but in *Staphisagria* children it comes from their sense of honor and in *Carcinosinum* children from their perfectionism and their urge to please other people. *Ignatia* children experience criticism as a personal failure. They always do their best to avoid making mistakes. If someone nevertheless finds fault, they feel like a failure. A reprimand or a harsh judgment from the teacher can make them literally ill. They find it difficult to come to terms with the insult. Exactly as with *Staphisagria* children, the sense of honor and wounded pride play a role.

If they've ever experienced something like this, they'll make sure they're prepared for it in the future. One of the possible ways that *Ignatia* children try to avoid criticism is by behaving childishly. Then they're taken less seriously and, therefore, less is expected of them. It's a bit like *Barium carbonicum* children, who feel inferior and "smaller" than the others, and thereby give an impression of childishness. Behind the childish behavior in *Ignatia* children, there's considerable sensitivity and pride. They know what they're worth and would like to show it ... if only people wouldn't criticize them!

Friendship

When *Ignatia* children do something, it's always with 100% commitment. This is also true for relationships. When they're young, they form friendships openly and straightforwardly. They believe that other children have the same high standards as they do. It's just not done to let down a friend! They're bound to be disappointed sooner or later because the perfect friendship doesn't exist on earth. The first time this happens, they're devastated. After that, they're more cautious about calling someone a friend. *Ignatia* children would like to protect themselves from injury.

When together with friendship there's also the matter of being in love, it gets a bit trickier. *Ignatia* boys and girls mostly don't flirt. Love is something solemn and should be forever. They'll do everything to make the relationship as perfect as possible and to protect it. If they're nevertheless betrayed or abandoned, they're inconsolable.

Hiding their grief

Ignatia is not for nothing the chief remedy for grief, especially lovesickness or the loss of a beloved person due to death. Everyone, including children, can suffer from a major loss, causing an "*Ignatia* state" that can be healed by *Ignatia*.

The reaction to grief is to withdraw, literally and figuratively. *Ignatia* children are very good at controlling their grief and covering it up so that no one will notice it. They can even laugh and make jokes after having just experienced something awful. Yet this "shell" is very fragile. If someone says something that moves them or reminds them of their troubles, they can suddenly and uncontrollably burst out weeping. When they're somewhat older, this weeping can sound hysterical — as if it's coming out of nowhere. Obviously the grief is there, but deeply hidden and suppressed.

It's best not to try and console *Ignatia* children at such times. They certainly want someone to be with them, but you should wait until they ask for consolation since they like to retain control!

Psychosomatic illnesses

Although *Ignatia* children are afraid of incurable illnesses, and quickly get the feeling that they have something dreadful, they're mostly spared serious physical illness. Many complaints such as coughing, voice loss, trembling muscles, and even paralysis are due to suppressed emotion. They can suppress their emotions so much that they virtually no longer feel anything. Obviously, this can lead in the long run to further physical symptoms. *Ignatia* invariably improves these complaints and brings emotional relief.

Physical symptoms

In the physical area, too, we see contradictory and changeable symptoms such as nausea that's improved by eating, emptiness in the stomach that's improved by fasting, and so on.

After grief or trouble, various different symptoms can arise, such as voice loss or paralysis but also sleeplessness and loss of appetite. *Ignatia* is one of the remedies for anorexia nervosa.

A typical symptom for *Ignatia* is sweating only on the face.

Food and Drink

Ignatia children love fruit (or reject it!), cheese, sour food, tomatoes, and bread. They can't tolerate cigarette or cigar smoke, and coffee worsens their symptoms.

The Kalium carbonicum Child

Potassium carbonate, Potash (K_2CO_3). Mineral remedy

"That's just right and proper!"

Origin

Kalium carbonicum is prescribed less often for children than for adults. It's always difficult to say whether a remedy is needed less in children or whether we just find it harder to recognize the remedy picture in children. The opposite is true, for example, for *Calcarea carbonica*, a remedy that is used more often for children than for adults. In children, we recognize the remedy picture mostly from the particular physical symptoms of *Kalium carbonicum*.

Kalium carbonicum is a compound of the chemical elements potassium (Latin: "kalium") and carbon. Potassium is one of the most common elements in the plant kingdom, and in ancient times this mineral was extracted from plant ash, potash. That's where the name "potassium" originally comes from. In the human body, it occurs especially in the cells. Carbon forms the basis of all organic compounds and is a special element. It is the stable foundation of all life on earth and constitutes the "scaffolding" of the human body.

Homeopathically, potassium stands for "sense of duty," a feeling of "That's right and proper." Carbon relates to the feeling of self-worth. Starting from these essences, we can clearly explain the overall picture of *Kalium carbonicum*.

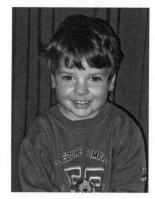

Kali-c.

Sober doers

The latest insights indicate that *Kalium* fits children who simply do what they have to and what they want to — spontaneously, without thinking about it much. In this way they make a pretty sober, "cool" impression. They're not concerned with attracting attention or giving others pleasure. It's not that they're unfeeling — they're definitely not that — yet they don't easily get worked up about other people's opinions. We find this kind of worry and fear more with *Calcarea carbonica* or *Calcarea silicata*. *Kalium carbonicum* children enjoy what they're doing and like busying themselves with practical things. They're willing to be told what to do by others since they don't have much fantasy or creativity of their own. On the other hand, they have good practical understanding. If they're shown how to do something, they'll copy it. They're doers — no words, just deeds. Doing puzzles, making things, helping their father repair something ... they're the best at that sort of thing. In this, they're similar to *Nux vomica* children, except that *Nux vomica* children are far more passionate, industrious, and touchy. *Kalium carbonicum* children don't get disturbed by others, unless they're being prevented from doing something. Their attitude to what they do is characterized by the notion: "You have to do what you have to do."

Secure foundation

The similarity with *Calcarea carbonica* children is that they need a secure foundation. They need to know where they stand. The family in which they grow up is very important for them and takes first place. *Kalium carbonicum* children are very sensitive to values and norms coming from their parents and will follow these closely in their own lives. They're real family types. Problems can occur if something is missing here, for example, if their father is absent due to separation, illness, or death, or if he's often away on business. *Kalium carbonicum* children need a strong father figure, since otherwise they lack a role model for their lives. This is obviously true for all kinds of children, but it's particularly important for these children. Exactly like *Graphites* children, they can become hard and stubborn and in the event of failure they can more quickly become unsettled. The difference from *Graphites* children is that *Kalium carbonicum* children derive their self-worth from their deeds, whereas *Graphites* children are still struggling with their identity.

Fixed standards – don't argue!

They have fixed standards and ideas. Once they know the rules, they'll normally stick to them but without the rigidity of *Cuprum* or the fanaticism of *Mercurius* children. No, they stick to the rules simply because that's right and proper. They follow the norms and values from their home without questioning. There's no doubt about it, even when they come across children at school with quite different norms and values. Indeed, this can have a positive effect on them since otherwise they might tend to become too rigid.

They're not particularly open to other opinions and they have difficulty putting themselves in someone else's shoes. It's also hard for them to explain to someone why they're thinking and behaving in this way. They haven't thought about it – they've simply learned to do things this way and that's it! Things are black and white, good or evil. They can't conceive of a middle way. The reality is obviously more complex but a lack of flexibility is one of the main problems with *Kalium carbonicum* children.

Inner sensitivity

On the outside, they're mostly calm and composed yet on the inside they can be struggling with various uncertainties, especially if there are grounds for this. They are not the kind of children, like *Calcarea carbonica*, who will make up problems. As mentioned above, they need a solid basis, a family in which they can place their trust. If this isn't available, they look for an alternative. This is their vulnerability. The fear of darkness and loneliness, which we also see with *Kalium carbonicum* children, symbolically represents the need for security. Small children like to be near their parents, want to hold their hand, and like being carried.

Uncertainty makes them nervous and can give them stomach problems. If they take fright – and this happens easily – they feel it in the stomach. "Fear in the stomach region" is a very characteristic symptom for this particular remedy. A further specific symptom is oversensitivity to touch. They can scarcely tolerate someone touching their feet. These seem to represent their foundation. If someone attacks their ideas or disregards their rules, they can easily become unsettled, and they want to avoid this by all possible means.

Emotions under control

Kalium carbonicum children are not quick to show their feelings. When they're small, they tend to behave shyly and cautiously in a strange place. At home, they feel fine and can express their feelings more easily. Yet if things are strained at home, there too they'll try to keep their emotions under control. On the inside, they can be seething with rage and will even dream about it. One of the typical dreams of *Kalium carbonicum* children is that they start a quarrel with someone close to them. What they aren't allowed to express — it's difficult for them to be angry with someone who they're dependent on — comes out at night in dreams.

Kalium carbonicum helps these children to once more become free and flexible, both with themselves and others. They learn that they are more important in themselves than for what they do and that they don't only need to act out of a sense of duty. They can be themselves again and make decisions from the heart.

Physical symptoms

It's the airways and the throat that are the most sensitive in *Kalium carbonicum* children. We often find difficulties in swallowing with very young children. The food remains stuck in the throat, which can make breathing difficult. We also see the feeling of suffocation in older children as well as asthma. In general, *Kalium carbonicums* feel the cold and are sensitive to changes in the weather. They should sit upright during an asthma attack, since lying down is impossible. If there's mucus in the lungs, they have difficulty coughing it up. The coughing often sounds dry.

A characteristic symptom for this remedy is for one ear to be red and warm.

The sensitivity is not just psychological but also physical — they're particularly sensitive to touch on the soles of the feet. The sensitivity to pain on the soles of the feet can be seen symbolically as the need for security, since we maintain contact with the earth through the soles of the feet.

A distended belly and painful hemorrhoids can also be an indication for this remedy, just as alternating constipation and diarrhea can be.

Typical for the *Kalium* type is the worsening of symptoms between 02:00 and 04:00 (2 and 4 a.m.).

Food and Drink

These children mostly have a desire for sweet things, especially sugar, although this doesn't agree with their digestive tract. They don't like soup and bread.

The Lac caninum Child

Dog's milk.

Animal remedy

"The Underdog: submissive"

Origin

Even around the time of Christ, the Roman writers Pliny and Dioscorides were familiar with the healing effect of dog's milk. They prescribed it to, among others, pregnant women, to induce birth and also as an antidote in cases of poisoning. It was not until the 19th century that *Lac caninum* was discovered afresh, this time by a homeopath, Dr. Reisig of New York. In a contemporary homeopathic journal, he described good results treating diphtheria. Due to his publications, other homeopathic doctors began to prescribe *Lac caninum* and — thanks to the remedy provings from that time — the remedy picture is very detailed.

In the last ten to fifteen years, the picture has become well-defined, including on the mental-emotional level, and we now have a clear idea of which type of child the remedy fits.

Accepting your place

Dogs evolved from wolves, and when we observe the life of these animals, we can begin to understand the children who need *Lac caninum*. The faithfulness of dogs is well-known, as is their devotion to their master. Dogs and wolves accept a hierarchy. You need to know and accept your place in the pack, even if you don't always agree with the behavior of those higher up the pecking order. So *Lac caninum* children respect authority.

When they're well treated by their parents and teachers, and their position is respected, they feel fine. They don't have problems with authority, as long as the authority figures are honest and just, and as long as they get recognition for what they do. But problems arise when someone oversteps the boundaries.

137

Self-Image

The self-image of *Lac caninum* children depends very much on the way they're treated, and this is their weak point. Basically, they attach a lot of importance to the opinions of the people who are in their eyes higher up, and they tend to play a submissive role.

This begins with their parents. They look up to them and give their best so as to be popular with them. If the parents and teachers positively support and respect these children, they'll grow up to be well-adjusted. But unfortunately, many parents and teachers never exercise authority properly. Abuse of power takes many forms and is often particularly subtle. It's not just a question of physical or verbal violence, but also of casual remarks with barely concealed disapproval and reproof. *Lac caninum* children are sensitive to just these kinds of signals, and accept the negative judgment of the other person as part of their own self-image.

Harassment and intimidation

Due to their submissive behavior, these children are liable to suffer harassment and intimidation at school, which makes them an easy target for children who are trying to increase their authority by humiliating others. The consequences of this intimidation can often be deep-reaching. Children who are harassed can completely lose their self-confidence. Even psychological disturbances from later in life can often be traced back to such experiences. Their self-image suffers lasting damage. It's especially important not just that the humiliation stops, but also that the children learn to stand up for themselves better. In this respect, *Lac caninum* gives these children valuable support.

Worthless

One of the expressions that *Lac caninum* children often use to express their feelings is: "I feel worthless." They feel inferior and believe that others look down on them. This already shows how negative their self-image is. They also accept someone else's judgment of their appearance only too easily. They rarely find themselves attractive. Instead, they frequently think of themselves as ugly or even repulsive. This can be traced back to a profound insult in the past, such

138

as sexual abuse or some other kind of violation where their personal boundaries were not respected. These children are generally obedient and only occasionally rebellious. They can obviously get angry, but a lot needs to happen for the anger to break out, since they mostly repress it. When the bottled-up anger is suddenly released, they behave like a dog gone wild. They go berserk due to everything that's been done to them. In a safe environment, such as the circle of the family, the anger can obviously break out more easily.

Physical symptoms

Lac caninum has a special relationship to the throat, to the female sex organs, and to the nervous system. Illnesses such as sore throats, diphtheria, and rheumatic complaints — for which the early homeopathic doctors prescribed the remedy — are still indications for it.

Very characteristic for all kinds of pain is that the side can change: headaches that start on the right switch to the left, and then back again to the right, or sore throats that wander from side to side, are strong hints for *Lac caninum*.

Oversensitivity of the nerves is very noticeable. This can lead to restlessness, mental over-stimulation, and exhaustion, and also to oversensitivity to touch. For example, *Lac caninum* children can't tolerate it when their fingers or limbs touch each other. The female sex organs are also very sensitive to touch. On the other hand, *Lac caninum* children can get a feeling of not touching the ground when they walk or not touching the bed that they're lying in, which can be thought of as a loss of feeling. Finally, the skin can show various symptoms such as inflammation and abscesses.

Food and Drink

The children often have a strong desire for milk and spicy food as well as pepper, cinnamon, and salt. They're reluctant to accept other drinks, even water. They don't like sweet things so much. It's noticeable that *Lac caninum* children are just as hungry after food as before — there's no feeling of fullness.

The Lachesis Child

Lachesis muta, Bushmaster snake
Animal remedy (Crotalidae family)

"Listen to me!"

Origin

In the Amazon jungle, the name of this snake is spoken with respect. The people there call it "surukuku" or "the bushmaster" — and not without reason. Every snake has its own particular territory. Small snakes mostly have a small territory, whereas large snakes like the Surukuku have a big one. Anything and anyone entering this area is viewed as an intruder. They're aggressive and will defend their territory, but can also be passionate in their love play! The South American temperament of the Surukuku is clearly recognizable in the remedy picture of *Lachesis*.

Constantin Hering – a German doctor and researcher, the founder of homeopathy in America – conducted the first remedy proving in 1828 with the venom of this huge snake (it can grow up to 12 feet, almost 4 meters, long!).

It gets the name "Lachesis" from Linnaeus, who named it after one of the three Greek goddesses of fate, the one who determines the length of the thread of life — that is, who decides how long we should live.

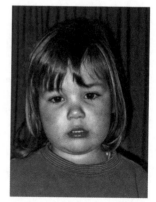

Lach.

Passion

Lachesis children are passionate by nature. They can be gushingly cheerful, warm-hearted, and loving, yet also explosive, furious, aggressive, and full of hate. They have an intense emotional life. As long as they're able to express their emotions, everything's alright. They need a lot of attention and love and are in their element when they get enough of this from their parents. Then we see warm-hearted and compassionate children. When someone has conquered their heart, they will go through hell and high water for this person. But it's important to first win their confidence. Before they open up, they need to be sure that people are well-meaning toward them. They have a special instinct for this and are particularly critical of others, which comes from their innate pride. Not for nothing are these snakes called "bushmaster": they have a dominant character and want everything to run according to their ideas. Straight from the cradle, they can rule the people around them with an almost hypnotic look! They need plenty of space and don't like to be cramped. This is symbolically represented by their reluctance to wear tight clothing round the neck (such as a turtle-neck sweater) or the waist.

Attention

A picture that we see in all snake remedies is the feeling of loneliness and of being abandoned. *Lachesis* shows this theme strongly. *Lachesis* children constantly need reassuring that they're loved, seen, and especially heard! As soon as they can speak, they demand attention for their stories. When they're small, they babble incessantly. This is how they like to express their emotions. They want to give vent to their feelings!

Yet if they get too little attention, and that will always be a subjective thing, then two things can happen: either they force people to give them attention — negative attention is also attention — or they withdraw into themselves. A remedy with a similar picture is the plant remedy *Hyoscyamus*.

A situation in which this character trait reveals itself clearly is when a sibling is born. Everyone's attention is suddenly concentrated on the newborn baby. *Lachesis* children then often feel deprived and it's this feeling that can lead to jealousy, which in turn leads to bad behavior to get the parents' attention and also to vent their feelings on the brother or sister.

A mother confided to me that she was very concerned about her 10-year old son. Since the birth of his younger brother, he had withdrawn increasingly into himself. When his little brother was playing with friends, he couldn't stop spoiling their game. When he shortly afterwards came down with a left-sided tonsillitis — one of the typical complaints of Lachesis — I took the opportunity to prescribe Lachesis. The tonsillitis was better within one day, the feeling of being discriminated against disappeared, and his original cheerfulness completely returned.

Strong intellect

Lachesis children usually have a powerful personality and a strong sense of reason. Thanks to their well-developed intuition, they grasp things quickly and can empathize well. At school and in other groups of children, they're often chosen to be the leader. They have a charismatic quality and can speak persuasively. Boys will tend to make use of their intellect, whereas girls will rather trust their feelings.

They also use their strong intellect to control their emotions. On the outside, they're calm, restrained children, but on the inside it's like a hurricane! For other people — including for the homeopathic doctor — they're difficult children to fathom, and it's not easy to recognize the Lachesis picture! Only when we appreciate the way in which open, demanding children can become intellectual and restrained is the remedy picture clear.

Big heart but easily hurt

In general, it's true for everyone that their greatest strength lies in their greatest vulnerability. While warm and empathetic, they're easily hurt by rejection. The saying: "When love turns to hate ..." certainly applies to this type of child. Even though they appear very intellectual, in fact they're ruled by their heart. The heart of the adult Lachesis is also the most sensitive organ when they become disturbed! They're immensely resentful of those who've abandoned them. And this feeling is easily aroused. It's as if they feel: "If they're not for me, they're against me." There's no happy medium. Any kind of hurt, an argument, or — when they're older — unrequited love, sits deep. Then they suffer from strong feelings of loneliness, jealousy, and suspicion. They prefer to bask in the warmth of oth-

ers, but they're also willing themselves to give affection. Love is what they love to feel most!
The homeopathic remedy *Lachesis* can help to reawaken this strength.

Physical symptoms

Most complaints affect the left side of the body. Therefore, *Lachesis* children often suffer from left-sided sore throats. The throat is one of the most sensitive parts of their body. Frequent symptoms are the sensation of a lump in the throat, difficulty swallowing, or left-sided tonsillitis. They can't tolerate the pressure of clothing round the neck, such as a turtleneck sweater, tie, or scarf.
They easily get cold and can't tolerate warmth either. They get headaches in the sun. The worst season for them is spring. Spring-time lethargy and hay fever are possible symptoms.
In general, they're evening people who feel worse on waking.
Lachesis children prefer sleeping on the right side, and can get complaints if they sleep on the left side.
They bruise easily and tend to get red-faced. They also suffer from migraine, ear infections (left), and asthma (especially when falling asleep and when angry).

Food and Drink

Pasta and piccalilli are their all-time favorite food, whereas they don't like bread. Older children can have a liking for coffee.

The Lithium metallicum Child

Lithium (Li). Mineral remedy

"Peter Pan — the boy who wouldn't grow up"

Origin

Lithium is the lightest solid element on earth, and occurs in various kinds of rock such as amblygonite, spodumene, lepidolite, petalite, and triphylite. The name comes from the Greek "lithos," which means stone. Due to its high energy density and low weight, lithium is used industrially, for example, to make batteries. It's also used in light-metal alloys. Lithium was originally prescribed as a remedy for gout. By chance, allopathic medicine discovered its effectiveness in treating manic-depressive illness, for which it's one of the chief remedies.

Lithium ranks third after hydrogen and helium in the Periodic Table. From homeopaths' study of the periodic table, the overview of all chemical remedies, we've discovered that there's a clear relationship between human development and the elements. *Hydrogen* corresponds to the unborn human – children who are floating between "higher spheres" and the earth. *Helium* corresponds to the fetus in the security and warmth of the womb. *Lithium* belongs to the first stage of life, the period in which the child gets to know its parents.

Crybaby

Lithium babies are often crybabies. Even as tiny newborn babies, they often don't feel comfortable in their own skin. On the other hand, obviously not all crybabies are automatically *Lithium* babies, although it's important to tell the homeopath about the crying. Helplessness, dependence, and the need to be looked after are all things that we see in older *Lithium* children, just as we also see rash and impulsive behavior. These children can become afraid for the slightest reason, and then the next moment they're completely careless, as if they hadn't seen the danger at all.

One symptom that also points to *Lithium* is "regression." This term is often used when children suddenly slip back a step in their devel-

144

opment. This might be, for example, the reappearance of thumb sucking or bed-wetting, although these stages were already over (*Pulsatilla* is also a well-known remedy for this). It's usually a profound event that causes this regressive behavior. You need a professional homeopath to prescribe for this!

Energetic and childish

In many ways, *Lithium* children can often still behave like small children, even when they're older. They're mostly open, spontaneous children who can be very cheerful. They often have a bubbly energy and can get really enthusiastic about things. They get down to their work with much fantasy and boldness. It's also no surprise that they get on well with small children, since this allows them to once again be the small child that they somehow still feel themselves to be: impulsive, carefree, and unrestrained.

Lithium children love physical activity such as running and cycling — sport in general is good for them. Exercise refreshes them when they're feeling a bit depressed. As long as they feel energized, and there are not too many obstacles in the way, they can achieve a lot. When they get actively involved in something, they're very tenacious and not easily distracted — certainly a valuable quality in the eyes of other people. And this recognition is something they really need. But even lithium batteries run out eventually ...

Mood swings

When something happens to curb their vitality or when their "battery" is simply empty, the mood of these children can change abruptly. The previously fun-loving *Lithium* children then become quiet, gloomy, and lost in thought. In their "up" phase, they can encounter the world uninhibitedly — but therein lies their vulnerability. Their inner child hasn't armed itself for the harsh reality of life: although the purity of a young child may be valuable, responsibility is nevertheless demanded of older children. It's exactly this demand that's difficult for *Lithium* children to meet — due to their past, on account of a lack of parental love and attention, or even due to excessive mollycoddling. If they could have their own way, they would remain forever a child. Their mood seesaws strongly

145

— for example, on top of the world for months and then sick at heart for months. Yet *Lithium* children can also switch moods rapidly. Small things can completely confuse them — they're so easily influenced.

In their own little world

In later life, *Lithium* children can still be struggling with typical childhood fears such as fear of the dark, fear of being alone, fear of strangers, and so on. They need support and will ask for it. They want to be taken care of by others, and don't want to have to stand on their own two feet. It's this feeling that explains why *Lithium* children in puberty easily become addicted to cigarettes, alcohol and drugs or gambling. They're looking for warmth and protection, and when they don't get these, they withdraw into their own world or look for some other source of satisfaction. With adults, they often have difficulties, unless these adults resemble their own parents. Most of all, they seek contact with children, animals, or nature in general. There they feel at home. In the grown-up world, they have to make decisions, which is difficult for them.

Physical symptoms

Lithium children feel "smaller" (younger) than they really are. In reality, they are indeed mostly smaller than other children of the same age. Growth disorders in the early years are an indication for *Lithium*.

When they don't feel well, their inner restlessness can lead to sleep disorders or even to complete sleeplessness. Muscle twitches can also occur in *Lithium* children, in the face as well as in the hands and feet. Hereditary eye complaints are often found in these children. The thyroid (over- and under-functioning) and the gut (constipation and diarrhea) are their weak points. We often also see skin complaints, ranging from eczema through herpes to psoriasis.

Food and Drink

Lithium children really like chocolate but don't always tolerate it well.

The Lithium phosphoricum Child

Lithium phosphate (Li_3PO_4). Mineral remedy

"Impulsive and changeable friendships"

Origin

This remedy is produced from a compound of lithium and phosphorus. It's one of the newer remedies that are used nowadays thanks to our knowledge of the periodic table, the overview of all chemical elements. *Lithium* and *Phosphorus* are both described separately in this book. *Lithium phosphoricum*, the remedy made by combining these two chemical substances, has qualities of each plus some of its own characteristics. It is especially interesting because it's one of the most important remedies for the treatment of Attention-Deficit Hyperactivity Disorder (ADHD).

Lithium fits children who throw themselves into things without thinking and who, due to uncertainty, are very changeable in their behavior and their mood. *Phosphorus* fits children for whom contacts, friendship, and communication are very important. It's this combination that gives rise to the picture described below.

Impulsive Contacts

The most striking symptoms of *Lithium phosphoricum* children, besides their openness and directness, are the longing for contact and the fickleness and impulsiveness with which they seek this contact. If they like someone, they just go up to the person without any shyness and ask, for example: "Do you want to be my girlfriend?" At such moments they will do everything possible to establish a relationship. The way in which they approach things is spontaneous and uncomplicated. Yet they're less concerned with how the other person experiences it – not all children react positively to such an invitation. They simply do whatever occurs to them at the time. They're not particularly loyal in their relationships and often have friendships that are quickly over. They've hardly got to know somebody when someone else arouses their interest. In this way, *Lithium phosphoricum* children are quick to switch friends. Apart from that, they love traveling and meeting new people. Everything is intense but not necessarily deep. When they're cheerful, they're very cheerful, and the same is true when they're worried about something! If they have a friend, they feel great, but the longing is profound when they're missing somebody.

This way of making contact is appropriate for very young children, but when they get stuck in such "childish" ways of behaving — and that's characteristic for *Lithium phosphoricum* children — this can lead to problems.

Changeable

Lithium phosphoricum children don't feel at all self-confident. This can be due to the situation at home or it can be caused by particular events in their lives, such as at school. Although they're eager for knowledge, they often lack self-confidence and inner balance. On the other hand, they're unimaginably sociable and are constantly looking for friends. That's where they seek protection. They just don't exactly know how to go about it and tend to throw themselves into a friendship "on the spur of the moment." This rash and impulsive behavior can, however, be completely misunderstood. Instead of receiving the recognition they're seeking, they're easily rejected. This rejection shakes them to the core and serves to reinforce their inner restlessness. They become ever more unsettled and go in search of recognition in new relationships.

Lithium phosphoricum helps them to recover their inner balance so that they're able to form more stable relationships and to develop more confidence in themselves and their intellectual abilities.

Attention-Deficit Hyperactivity Disorder (ADHD)

As already mentioned, *Lithium phosphoricum* seems to be one of the most important homeopathic remedies for hyperactivity. Additional remedies relevant here are *Tuberculinum*, *Medorrhinum*, *Saccharum*, and *Belladonna*.

Lithium phosphoricum helps when the overall picture of the child is consistent. The child is open, curious, and sympathetic. Contact is

148

made in an impulsive, childish way. If these symptoms are not present, it's worth considering another remedy.

Physical symptoms

Lithium phosphoricum children can develop various physical symptoms that also affect *Lithium* or *Phosphorus* children.

The *Lithium* theme of "remaining a child" turns up again as delayed growth, which can, however, be due to under-functioning of the thyroid gland. Together with prescribing *Lithium phosphoricum*, supplementing with thyroid hormone can be necessary.

The complaints occur mostly on the right side and are worsened by movement.

Lithium phosphoricum children are often overly sensitive to cats, smells, and wool. They have an increased tendency to bleed, which shows up as mild nosebleeds or bruises. Besides that, their airways are sensitive: they can get bronchitis, asthma, and various infections, often accompanied by swollen glands. Similarly, the stomach and gut are very sensitive. Particularly at night, they suffer from nausea, vomiting, and diarrhea, caused by chocolate and fruit, among other things.

Food and Drink

Exactly like *Phosphorus* children, they mostly have a strong desire for cold drinks and for fish. Besides that, they often have a preference for spicy food, salt, ice cream, chicken, and chocolate. There can also be a dislike of salt and fish. As mentioned above, they don't always tolerate chocolate and fruit well.

The Lycopodium Child

Lycopodium clavatum, Stag's-horn Clubmoss, Ground Pine

Plant remedy (Lycopodiaceae family)

"Internally powerful"

Origin

The Lycopodiaceae family is one of the oldest on earth. Millions of years ago, this family produced enormous plants up to 130 feet (40 meters) high with an average diameter of six feet (two meters). It's especially from thess plants that coal formed. Clubmoss — the spores of which are used to make the remedy *Lycopodium* — is, however, a moss-like herb with a creeping stem and branches about 5 inches (12 cm) high, from which spore cones develop.

The striking contrast between the once so powerful plant and its current stature is something we see reflected in the character of *Lycopodium* children. We can clearly see the idea of hidden greatness in the remedy picture of *Lycopodium*. The spores of this plant are used in the theatre and in pyrotechnics to produce fire. So they're very powerful and courageous!

In North America, one of the places where this plant grows, *Lycopodium* was used by the Blackfoot Indians to stop bleeding, heal

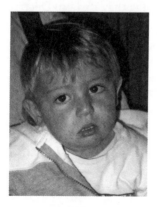
Lyc.

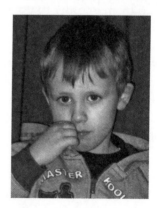
Lyc.

wounds, and induce perspiration. Conventional medicine of the 18th century used *Lycopodium* as a filler to complement other medicinal herbs. At that time, it was assumed that the plant didn't have any healing effect of its own. This view changed when Hahnemann homeopathically ground, diluted, and succussed it. As soon as it's made into a homeopathic remedy, *Lycopodium* is an unsurpassed medicine, especially in high potencies.

Sensitive to hierarchies

The character of *Lycopodium* children is rather like that of a wolf. The scientific name *"Lycopodium"* -- which is composed of the Greek words "lycos" (wolf) and "pos" (foot) -- was certainly not chosen at random. The common name "Wolfpaw clubmoss" comes from this. In a pack of wolves, there is a strict hierarchy. Each wolf attempts to climb the ladder, but must sooner or later yield to a stronger wolf. This pattern is something we also find with *Lycopodium* children, who will try even as small children to enlarge their own territory. As long as they don't encounter any stiff resistance, they'll continually expand the boundaries of their territory. So we can find that even a young *Lycopodium* child has already become the "head" of the family. But if there's just one person in the family — whether it be father, mother, brother, or sister — with a stronger character, the *Lycopodium* child will accept that person as the leader or "top dog." Yet they don't give up so easily. They constantly challenge the people around them in order to test out how far they can go. Deep inside, they know that they are powerful and strong, but they're forced to bow to the superior strength and power of the top dog. *Lycopodium* children demand that their parents and teachers behave in a careful and transparent way. They thrive best in a hierarchical atmosphere in which authority rests on clearly defined and real abilities.

Intellectuals

Many *Lycopodium* children are intellectually orientated, which doesn't mean they're no good at sport. On the contrary! Whatever they do, they try to do it as well as possible. They're very ambitious and want to be the best in everything. Yet they feel most at home with things intellectual. They're generally precocious, although they only undertake something when they're certain they can do it. As small children, they don't babble, but instead they only speak when they can articulate complete sentences! They obviously want to earn the recognition that they need — which is a lot. At the appropriate time, they also need clear explanations of what's allowed and what won't be tolerated.

They're easy to get along with and are very kind and friendly. At school, for example, the teacher won't understand when you try to explain how difficult your child is at home. In the classroom, these children are always keen and set an example to all. But when it happens that *Lycopodium* children feel at school as they do at home, the teacher will be confronted with the other side of this strong personality. Especially as adolescents, they take a critical view of their teachers. Only a handful of teachers will be able to live up to their standards — and they'll put these on a pedestal. They can express their contempt for a teacher they don't approve of very bluntly: "Idiot." When they know better than the teacher, they don't keep their opinion to themselves.

Ambitious children

The image of the mountain climber is often used to characterize *Lycopodium* children. They want to climb up and up, ever closer to the summit. This is especially true for intellectual achievements and their position in the social hierarchy. At the same time, they want to have everything under control, and they find it hard to trust others. As long as they're in control of the situation, everything's OK. But if they suddenly find themselves confronted with new challenges that they haven't bargained for, things can go wrong, since their self-confidence is a weak point. Inside, they're plagued by doubt as to whether they'll be able to reach the goal they've set themselves: "The higher they go, the harder they fall." They always want to get to the top, although they become anxious when they look back and realize how far they've come.

Their way of getting a grip on this anxiety is to prepare perfectly. *Lycopodium* children always try to cover themselves. If they have an examination, they try to learn everything so as to pass with flying colors. But if there's a question about something they're not sure of, they can panic. They want to avoid this at all costs.

King of their small kingdom

When *Lycopodium* children are settled, they can certainly be charming and obliging. They come across as open and docile, and in everything they do, they have a clear idea of what they want. Nevertheless, they exhibit a slight reserve, since deep inside a lingering doubt remains.

In an environment they know — such as at home, with friends, or in their school class — they're the "boss" and feel themselves superior to the others. When they notice that people are looking up to them, their self-confidence grows and can become a kind of arrogance. Children who, in their own way, have problems with "power" will likely find it difficult to get along with *Lycopodium* children, since there can only be one king!

Obedient or boastful

When *Lycopodium* children don't feel well, they can try to hide the feeling of uncertainty in two ways. One way is to avoid taking on any responsibility, thereby becoming helpless, frightened, and obedient, meanwhile flattering the stronger person. The other way is to cover up their uncertainty in a display of swaggering bravura, often with a dictatorial touch — and if words aren't enough, they can resort to swearing, hitting, and kicking. Obviously, neither of these approaches solves the problem. The solution is, as always, somewhere in the middle.

If they listen to their inner voice and learn to trust in their abilities, they can act from a position of strength once more. It can, however, be necessary to work through old hurts they might have experienced — for example, due to a strict father. *Lycopodium* can support this process and help the children to be themselves again.

Physical symptoms

Lycopodium children are often really grumpy in the morning. It's best to leave them alone for a while after they wake up, although a dose of *Lycopodium* can work wonders. Between 16:00 and 20:00 (4 and 8 p.m.), they also don't feel so good, especially when they're ill too. Many complaints occur on the right side or affect organs on the right. So the liver is one of the most sensitive organs for *Lycopodium*

153

children. In Chinese medicine, liver complaints indicate unresolved anger, a problem that occurs often with *Lycopodium* children.

Another sensitive organ is the gut. Exactly as they "puff" themselves up to compensate for their sense of powerlessness, so as to appear bigger, the gut also has a tendency to retain air, leading to distention of the abdomen. Belching and breaking wind provide relief for them. With their bowel movements, it's noticeable that the stool is initially hard and difficult to expel, whereas the final portion is thin and soft.

Small children sometimes have cradle cap, milk crust, seborrheic eczema, or seborrheic dermatitis. In older children, we often see pimples, dandruff, and warts on the hands.

In countries where homeopathy is also used in hospitals, such as India, *Lycopodium* is one of the most important remedies for the early stages of a lung infection.

Food and Drink

Lycopodium children can have a very changeable appetite — sometimes a lack of appetite then ravenous hunger. It's best if they eat small amounts regularly. They have a strong desire for sweet things although these tend to worsen the flatulence.

The Magnesium carbonicum Child

Magnesium carbonate (MgCO₃)

Mineral remedy

"Problems with the father figure"

Father figure

Magnesium carbonicum children have the same fears as all other *Magnesium* children, although everything in their lives revolves around the father figure. This can concern an argument with the father or it can be about the (threatened) loss of the father.

We often see this picture in children whose parents are separated, rather like the picture of *Magnesium muriaticum*. *Magnesium carbonicum* children generally react in the same way as *Magnesium muriaticum* children, either with adaptation or aggression. Sometimes these two reactions alternate.

The difference between the pictures of *Magnesium muriaticum* and *Magnesium carbonicum* is that *Magnesium muriaticum* is concerned primarily with protection, attention, and care (to do with the mother), whereas in *Magnesium carbonicum* the central themes are recognition and respect (to do with the father).

Self-Worth

The father figure (Carbon) has a decisive influence on the development of our sense of self-worth. The ideal father affirms us in what we do and encourages us to act in the outside world so that we can assume our rightful place there.

Magnesium relates to the time when the child is making contact with others and taking up his place in the world. The child already has a certain amount of self-confidence but needs to learn how to behave with other people, how to make contact, and how to maintain relationships.

Magnesium carbonicum children experience problems establishing a relationship with the father figure. In addition, *Magnesium* has to do with aggression — the remedy corresponds to the phase in which

Magnesium carbonate ($MgCO_3$)

children are busy consolidating their own "territory." So there are several ways in which a *Magnesium carbonicum* state can arise.

Aggression

If a father is too aggressive, he can overstep his children's boundaries with his aggression. He fails to respect their territory, and his strength forces them to react. Children long for the approval of their father and will try first and foremost to meet his wishes. How the children react depends on their character, the reaction of the father, and the reactions of the other family members. Problems arising here can be very complex and can often only be overcome by working with the family as a group (family therapy). Well-known patterns of reaction include: adapting, trying to avoid conflicts, ensuring that the father doesn't get angry, appeasing. Or just the opposite: the child becomes aggressive and provokes conflict in order to wring some respect and recognition from the father and to clearly mark the boundaries. The picture of aggression is the most well-known for *Magnesium carbonicum*: rather "disgusted," difficult, aggressive children, always stirring up trouble.

A father who is almost never angry can cause exactly the same problems. The children then don't know where they are with him. They want recognition and respect, yet an overly weak father doesn't respect himself enough and so can't give the children sufficient recognition. In this case too, the children can react aggressively so as to exact some respect. Or they copy the father's behavior by avoiding conflict.

Peacemaker

The picture of the "peacemaker" is at least as important as that of the overly aggressive child. It is, however, not so easy to recognize, since the behavior of these children is less problematic for other people. Yet for the child, it's very important that this pattern is recognized early and the appropriate treatment given, since the repressed aggression can really damage the child, mentally as well as physically. Moreover, this opens the door to behavior that violates these children, as they never get angry. If the problems aren't solved at a young age, we see the patterns being repeated in later life — for example, in the relationship with a partner or at work. The feeling of self-worth in both types of children is ruined. They're mostly missing a healthy sense of self-respect and quickly get the impression that they're undervalued. With parents who are constantly quarreling, these children can even get the impression that they are the subject of the parents' arguments — that the parents want to divorce and abandon the children, because they're worthless after all!

Orphans

James Tyler Kent, one of the most famous American homeopaths, mentions *Magnesium carbonicum* as the primary remedy for orphans. In the meantime, we've found that there are a few remedies that are maybe even better for the "orphaned child," namely *Glechoma hederacea* (ground ivy or Creeping Charlie) and *Oxalicum acidum* (oxalic acid). In German, a traditional name for ground ivy is "little orphan child"! *Oxalicum acidum* fits best children who have been adopted.

When the aggression comes from the father figure, we must think of *Magnesium carbonicum*. In the old orphanages, the children were often brought up very strictly, with the severe teachers taking on the role of the violent father. The children either become rebellious and aggressive or they repress their anger. In both cases, we see a typical *Magnesium carbonicum* picture.

Magnesium carbonicum can help these children to let go of old patterns of behavior, to work through their anger towards the father figure, and to regain a feeling of self-worth. In the clinic, we can see that aggressive children become calmer and can deal with their anger more appropriately, whereas the "peacemakers" become surer of themselves, more able to take on conflicts, and learn how to stake out their boundaries.

Physical symptoms

As we notice with all *Magnesium* compounds, *Magnesium carbonicum* children often have digestive complaints (for example, cramps, constipation or diarrhea, sour stool). They also often suffer from neuralgia, especially in the jaw.

The Magnesium muriaticum Child

Magnesium chloride (MgCl₂). Mineral remedy

"Don't abandon me!"

Origin

In addition to the metal magnesium, *Magnesium muriaticum* also consists of chloride. It's gradually become clear to us homeopaths that chloride relates to the mother figure, which represents care and attention. We can find these themes in various forms in the remedy picture of *Magnesium muriaticum*. Although the remedy is not suited to self-medication, it is indeed true that almost all children (and adults) who have witnessed the separation of their parents need this remedy to cope with the grief, anger, and fear of abandonment. A prescription for this remedy can help even if the child doesn't necessarily correspond to the type – this is, by the way, true for most homeopathic remedies. The situation or the experience can be sufficient if the corresponding emotions are clearly present.

Loss of care and attention

Magnesium muriaticum is worth considering for anyone who has experienced the separation or loss of their parents and hasn't been able to work through the consequences. The main thing here is the (threatened) loss of care, the sense of no longer being looked after and cared for. In our society, these characteristics are attributed primarily to the mother.

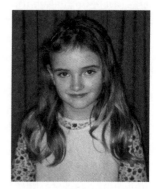

Mag-m.

Magnesium muriaticum children are mostly peace-loving characters. They have at some time experienced a separation or a family quarrel, which made them very afraid of arguments or violence afterwards. They often have an unconscious fear of losing someone again. They then can't tolerate any arguments with or between the people around them, and they become known as peacemakers. *Magnesium muriaticum* can — along with good psychological care — help them to work through the trauma and to once again become confident in their relationships. They learn to allow themselves to be angry when the situation demands it.

Peace or dispute?

To avoid the threatened loss, the children can react in two different ways. One group fits in and tries everything to keep the peace, even going so far as to repress their feelings. The other group tries to hold on to or restore the relationship by force. In the first case, *Magnesium muriaticum* children become the typical "peacemakers," children who are always trying to settle disputes and who feel distinctly unwell when they don't achieve this. They're also usually sensitive to injustice. On the other hand, the children who react forcefully do so in order to attract attention and to function as a lightning conductor for the arguments in the family. The way they do this can be vehement since the anger in *Magnesium muriaticum* children is very strong.

Physical symptoms

Magnesium muriaticum has a specific relationship to the liver. It is one of the remedies for inflammation of the liver when no particular cause can be found. Therefore, they can't tolerate heavy food, fat, and milk. They easily get diarrhea, especially after drinking milk. They can also suffer from headaches as a result of disturbed liver function.

They often wake up tired, since they aren't refreshed by sleep. Only in the course of the day do they begin to feel better.

Food and Drink

These children love sweet things and vegetables. They can't tolerate milk and heavy, fatty food.

The Magnesium phosphoricum Child

Magnesium phosphate (MgHPO₄)

Magnesium phosphate (MgHPO$_4$)

Mineral remedy

"Fear of losing contact"

Magnesium compounds

Magnesium muriaticum is related to the mother-child relationship, *Magnesium carbonicum* to the father-child relationship, and *Magnesium phosphoricum* to the relationships with siblings and friends.

The general *Magnesium* themes are aggression (to mark out your own territory) or the exact opposite, namely the tendency to avoid conflicts and arguments, as well as a fear of loss.

Sensitive

Phosphorus is about social contacts in general. Behind the strong need for communication, there's a fear of being alone. Without relationships, they feel themselves to be "alone on a desert island." *Phosphorus* represents relationships to siblings and friends. So with *Magnesium phosphoricum* children, we see problems in this area.

Yet *Phosphorus* also has other characteristics that we can read about in the remedy picture of *Phosphorus*. They're mostly sensitive, sympathetic, and empathetic children, who can sense what's going on in their fellow human beings. They can certainly be angry, but it's usually short-lived and doesn't go deep. They find it hard to endure long-term tension. *Magnesium phosphoricum* children are even more sensitive where moods and arguments are concerned.

Problems with the brother or sister

A *Magnesium phosphoricum* picture can arise in young children due to problems with the siblings. The brother or sister is quarrelsome and influences the atmosphere in the family by their aggressive behavior. A *Magnesium phosphoricum* child will react by behaving calmly or trying to settle the conflict and defuse the tension. If *Magnesium phos-*

phoricum children are drawn into the dispute, however, they can also show aggressive behavior.

A further situation in which a *Magnesium phosphoricum* picture can arise is a family in which the parents argue a lot. *Magnesium phosphoricum* children fear that the parents will separate, the family break up, and that they'll then lose contact with the family members.

Quarrels with a friend

Magnesium phosphoricum children are sensitive in terms of friendships. They have a need for friends and will do anything to make and maintain friendships. They're afraid of losing their friends and not having any relationships any more. If they have a quarrel with a friend, they can react in one of two ways. They either try to repress their own anger "for the sake of peace and quiet," or they behave angrily and aggressively. An unspoken conflict with a friend can generate a *Magnesium phosphoricum* picture with all its complaints. The picture is generally only clear when physical symptoms also arise.

Physical symptoms

Magnesium phosphoricum children mostly feel the cold and react sensitively to thunderstorms. They also suffer from neuralgia in the face or muscle cramps that can occur in various parts of the body. Writer's cramp or finger cramps in pianists fit this remedy. The pains can be burning.

Abdominal cramps, in which the child is relieved by pressure, a hot-water bottle, or by bending forwards, are characteristic for *Magnesium phosphoricum*. The same cramps can occur during menstruation in girls.

Food and Drink

Magnesium phosphoricum children generally love fish and cold drinks as well as tangy and salty food. On the other hand, they can dislike salt and fish.

The Manganum metallicum Child

Manganese, black magnesia (Mn). Mineral remedy

"Helpful in the background"

Origin

Manganese was discovered in 1774. Its name is derived, exactly like magnesium, from the area Magnesia in the Greek province of Thessaly. After iron, manganese is the most frequently occurring heavy metal in the earth's crust. In the periodic table, the overview of all chemical elements, it comes between chromium and iron (*Ferrum*). The metal has several unusual characteristics, which are crucially important for the effect of the homeopathic remedy made from this metal. It can form various compounds, showing a changeable number of electrons. Most elements have a fixed number of electrons, and a few elements — the noble gases — don't form any compounds at all. Thanks to this characteristic, manganese can be used in multiple ways and possesses a rich color spectrum, depending on which substances it bonds with.

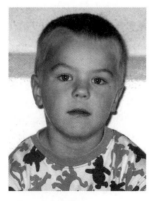
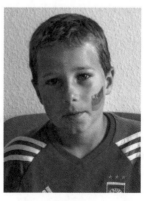

Mang. *Mang-p.*

Industry makes good use of manganese in steel alloys, which thereby become harder, more flexible and less fragile, as well as being easier to roll. Many pigments also contain manganese.

In our body, manganese plays an important role as an activator of enzymes, hormones, and vitamins, as well as in the formation of connective tissue and bone growth.

In conclusion, we can say that manganese, despite not playing a leading role, is nevertheless essential and plays a key background role ensuring that things run smoothly.

Obliging

Manganum children support others and like to be helpful to them. They are generally friendly children who tend to take a back seat in favor of other people. They fit in easily, and are in this respect like *Carcinosinum* children. Even small children needing this remedy show this characteristic. They are very sensitive and take on the worries of their parents. They like being complimented, since this is the reward that they're longing for. In this respect, they're similar to other metals: they're after recognition for good performance. But this can become compulsive. They have to help out, otherwise they feel unsettled. Only when they've been assured that they did something well can they settle down. They need that confirmation.

Another aspect is learning. They like learning and love to teach things to other children. Therefore, they don't necessarily experience criticism as negative, as long as it's constructive.

Physical symptoms

Manganum children react sensitively to damp cold. One of the most striking complaints is earache, caused by cold wind. When the wind is stronger than normal or when the air gets colder, they have to cover their ears.

Other complaints that we regularly see in *Manganum* children are diabetes mellitus and various neurological symptoms such as Tourette's syndrome (a neuropsychiatric illness characterized by tics). Hoarseness, cartilage complaints (cartilage tissue contains manganese), especially in the knee joint, as well as various skin diseases, including psoriasis, are also found.

163

Food and Drink

Just like *Ferrum* children, they either love or hate tomatoes. Tomatoes often disagree with them! They also can't tolerate cold food well, such as ice cream.

The Medorrhinum Child

Gonorrhea nosode

"Likeable, restless, and sometimes wild"

Origin

Medorrhinum is a deep and indispensable remedy. It's prescribed especially often for children, even for newborn babies. *Medorrhinum* is one of the nosodes — exactly like *Carcinosinum*, *Psorinum*, and *Tuberculinum* — which are remedies made from disease agents or products. Over one hundred years ago, homeopaths already knew that much disease could be traced back to the illnesses of the parents or their ancestors, which can still cause problems many generations later. The illnesses known at that time to cause complaints in the descendants were tuberculosis, gonorrhea, syphilis, scabies, and cancer. Since at that time there was no known medicine able to cure these illnesses, homeopathic doctors decided to make homeopathic remedies directly from the disease products. This was possible and harmless since, when preparing a homeopathic substance, not a single molecule of the original substance remains, due to the very high dilution used. Therefore, nosodes don't contain any germs. The Pasteur Institute in France recently confirmed this once

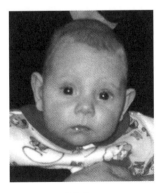
Med.

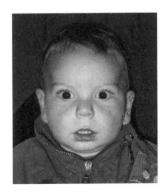
Med.

165

again. Even viruses and prions can't survive the production process. The remedy retains only the power to cure, without the harmful
effect!
Following this procedure, *Medorrhinum* is made from gonococcus,
the bacteria that causes gonorrhea (clap).

Seagoing ancestors

Gonorrhea (clap) is a sexually transmitted disease that's still common today, but in the past there were real epidemics of it. It spread
right round the world aboard ship, and almost every sailor was
infected with it. *Medorrhinum* is, therefore, a remedy that we still frequently need to completely heal a child.
Although we now have a good picture of the mental symptoms of
Medorrhinum, it's the physical complaints that give us the clearest
hints. Children who need *Medorrhinum* don't necessarily have to fit
the type. *Medorrhinum* is a remedy that is frequently needed at some
point during the healing process.

Complaints right from birth

Medorrhinum children often have complaints from birth onwards.
Colds in newborn babies, sometimes asthma (from which they get
relief in the knee-elbow position) and stubborn diaper rash are the
characteristic symptoms that point to a child needing *Medorrhinum*
— especially when all three symptoms occur together.
The symptoms can be mild as well as intense. Dr. Arij Vrijlandt, who
until his death ten years ago was the doyen of the homeopathic
doctors in the Netherlands, was once asked for help in a hospital.
A newborn baby had an apparently fatal metabolic disorder. Dr.
Vrijlandt could only find a single hint: the baby clearly preferred
the knee-elbow position (like a Muslim at prayer). For this reason,
he prescribed *Medorrhinum*, following which the baby's condition
improved markedly.

Likeable and tense

Typical *Medorrhinum* children are likeable, very sympathetic, and
crazy about animals. They love nature, plants, and trees, and have
a sense of beauty. They can react very emotionally, and even funny

or beautiful things can make them cry. In this respect, they're similar to *Phosphorus* children, although there's frequently a certain tension noticeable in them, which we can often see in their face — as if they're having to repress something or to get a grip on themselves in order to appear friendly (for example, by a forced smile).

Restlessness and moodiness

Their mood can change suddenly. For example, they can stroke the cat lovingly one moment and the next moment suddenly pinch its tail rather too aggressively. They feel an inner disquiet that older children describe as like having an engine running inside them that they can't turn off. When they can't find an outlet for this, they can become hyperactive.

If they're busy with something, they're always driven and in a rush. They only relax when everything's finished. They can't bear coming too late. It's as if the devil were hard on their heels!

Fear of the unknown

Everything lying ahead of them fills them with disquiet, a kind of anxiety. How will it go? What could possibly happen? They're always afraid that something will go wrong. Yet when you ask them why, they can't give you an answer. It's simply an inner feeling; there's no particular reason.

We can recognize the remedy in small children by, among other things, fear of the dark, a stuffed up nose, and a desire for ice cream. They also run around with an open mouth due to their blocked nose. They like to bite their fingernails and even their toenails! If the remedy is indicated, the inner disquiet disappears and the children can settle down.

Physical symptoms

Whether or not by chance, *Medorrhinum* children certainly feel better by the sea, and many of their complaints can disappear there. Asthma that improves in the sea air indicates *Medorrhinum*. It's striking that damp weather often improves their complaints, although cold dampness can cause them problems.

Medorrhinum children are real night owls. They can wake up at night and start playing, as they have the feeling that the new day has already started.

Allergies and inflammation affect many *Medorrhinum* children. The airways are often very sensitive, as are the mucous membranes of the nose and throat. They often get sinusitis. The phlegm gets stuck, so in the ears there can be temporary deafness, and the stuffed up nose impairs the sense of smell and taste.

Problems with the urinary tract in children are often an indication for *Medorrhinum*. During a bladder infection, the urine can be burning. The children often suffer from constipation. They frequently get eye infections, especially as newborns.

Further important symptoms in children are nail-biting, delayed growth, and a waxy, pale face.

Medorrhinum can remove a disturbance that has sometimes been in a family for generations, leading in many cases to a full cure.

Food and Drink

Medorrhinum children crave oranges, green apples, and juicy fruit. They can have a desire for lemons, raw onions, sweet things, salty things, fat, and ice cream. Here too we see extremes: from very healthy to very unhealthy.

There is often an aversion to slimy food.

Medorrhinum in the Clinic

Jost and his boils

The reason why Jost and his mother came to see me was his boils. He was twelve years old at the time and had been suffering from boils for the last four years. They appeared at different places on his body, were painful and accompanied by swollen glands. What's more, he had been given a diagnosis of asthma. He had regularly had impetigo on the mouth and chin and suffered from frequent ear infections. Jost also had complaints on going to sleep. When he was somewhat younger, he often played at night. He slept in the characteristic knee-elbow position.

His mother explained how he was always active and cheerful, and that he had difficulty doing things calmly. When he was ill, he became awkward and would kick things and look for a fight. His concentration deteriorated and he became forgetful.

As I listened to this, the decision for *Medorrhinum* became clearer and clearer. When his mother confirmed that Jost mostly felt better when they were at the seaside, I gave him a dose of *Medorrhinum*.

Six weeks later, the boils had disappeared, he was less short of breath, and he had become more lively. As time went by, Jost became calmer and fell asleep more easily. He continued to receive a dose of *Medorrhinum* 1,000c (1M) approximately every six weeks. After 9 months, his condition had improved so much that we decided to see each other only if his health deteriorated again.

Jochen: eczema and coughing

Jochen came for the first time when he was two years old. He had many problems with sore skin, eczema, and itching. When he was even younger, he had regularly had diaper rash. At night he coughed constantly. He could "bark" endlessly, and his breathing would sometimes make a whistling sound, especially when the weather was cold and damp.

During his first year, he had cried almost every night. Jochen too slept in the knee-elbow position.

He was a lively, mischievous little fellow. When he had the chance, he climbed over everything. He was curious but his concentration

169

was not good, and he could be unbelievably bad-tempered, especially when he was being held. His love of animals was noticeable. The whole thing, the illnesses, and also the character indicated *Medorrhinum*. I gave him *Medorrhinum* a few times. His complaints improved rapidly and he became calmer. When I saw him two years later, he no longer had any problems.

The Mercurius Child

Mercury (Hydrargyrum, Hg)

Mineral remedy

"Who's not for me is against me"

Origin

Mercurius – named after the Roman god of trade and the planet of the same name – is called "quicksilver" due to its form and color. In Hahnemann's time (in the second half of the 18th century and the first half of the 19th century), quicksilver was frequently used in conventional medicine for, among other things, the treatment of syphilis. Hahnemann, who was not only a doctor but also a great chemist, decided to try and find a compound that was less damaging, since the consequences of a dose of quicksilver were often worse than the illness for which it was prescribed. His discovery, *Mercurius solubilis Hahnemanni*, was quickly picked up by the conventional doctors. When he discovered homeopathy, he began to search for the purest form of *Mercurius*, a form with as little contamination from other elements as possible. This pure form of *Mercurius* he called *Mercurius vivus* (the official name at that time was "*Hydrargyrum purum*"), "living quicksilver," due to its fluid, mobile character at room temperature.

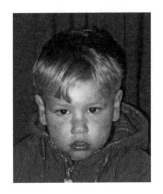

Merc.

Living thermometer

In homeopathy, *Mercurius* people are called "living thermometers," since they react to temperature changes just as sensitively as a thermometer. It's no accident that, due to its quick reaction to temperature changes, quicksilver is used in thermometers. It expands on warmth and contracts on cold. Children who need *Mercurius* tolerate both warmth and cold poorly.

171

When a thermometer breaks and the quicksilver flows out, it immediately forms tiny drops. Although it's fluid, it doesn't wet things and doesn't stick to anything. It seems to be very gentle, yet it contains enormous inner power. It can even completely dissolve gold, among other things!

Quicksilver is the most important element in amalgam, the metal alloy that's still used for dental fillings. It's also used to manufacture explosives! We can find many of these characteristics in the remedy picture of *Mercurius*.

A strong will and an independent opinion

We often find *Mercurius* and *Aurum* children in positions of leadership. Even at an early age, they demonstrate a strong will. They can only accept it with difficulty when things don't work out as they imagined. They can be very friendly and submissive, but they expect consistent behavior from their parents and teachers. *Mercurius* children have a particularly fixed opinion about what is right and proper, and what is not. If a particular pattern has established itself in their upbringing, it becomes very difficult to change it. They are very fixed and they think in black and white. The positive side of this is that they know where they stand and that, once they've accepted a rule, they don't easily break it. However, when something is arranged that can't be carried out as planned, it's very hard to make that clear to them. An agreement is an agreement! It takes real skill to give these children, who would rather just take over everything, the feeling that they themselves can decide about things. This means in practice that deviations from the norm need to be explained so that they understand why it's different this time. To simply force the child can turn out to be counterproductive, as they then become rebellious.

Right and wrong

Mercurius children have their own clear ideas about what's good and what's bad. Here too the upbringing is crucial. If they have an upbringing with clear rules and norms, this stays with them for the rest of their lives. If at home there are no clear rules, they make their own and stick to them. They're very sensitive where justice is concerned, yet here too they use their own norms and values when judging a situation. This is different from *Staphisagria* children, who generally react sensitively to the way people get on with one another, and who can sense whether this is based on respect. For *Mercurius* children, this might imply for example that they are furious when someone cycles on the footpath, even if no one is endangered. Exactly like *Cuprum* children, they're very good "police," who radiate even more of a sense of authority when they're feeling well. Yet they don't find it acceptable when they themselves — in their eyes — are not treated well, for example by the teacher.

Rage and inner restlessness

They can get furious when things don't go as they wish, when someone puts obstacles in their way, or when they feel disadvantaged by someone. This can be something that is, in the eyes of other people, completely unimportant. It's important that they have some way of calming down. An unjustified penalty can be the worst thing imaginable for them! When they can't get rid of their rage, they get nervous and restless, shake (with rage), and their voice starts to quiver. The explosion comes sooner or later, or else they get physically ill.

Everyone's against me!

Mercurius children like to have everything under control. When something interesting catches the eye of small *Mercurius* children, they want to grab hold of it straightaway. They want to be completely in charge of things. This means they can easily get into conflict with authority. As long as the authority figures act consistently, there's no problem, but when they deviate, they're sure to have difficulty with *Mercurius* children. The children react rebelliously and try to fight the "injustice." In this phase, they see potential enemies everywhere, as if to say: "Who's not for me is against me." It's not easy to get along with *Mercurius* children when they're like this, as they can interpret every word wrongly.

As long as they succeed in fighting for what they want, they're strong, but when they get the feeling that they're powerless, they start doubting themselves and their strength turns to weakness. Instead of the strong personalities that they basically possess, we then see nervous, stuttering, weak children with too little self-confidence.

It requires great commitment and empathy on the part of the parents to find the right balance between freedom and boundaries for these children, but it's certainly worth it. When they know where they stand, and they're allowed a certain freedom of action, they can develop into strong-willed people with enormous strength. These are the future leaders.

Physical symptoms

Mercurius has, along with sensitivity to warmth and cold, several characteristic symptoms. One of these is a copious flow of saliva, especially at night, which can be accompanied by a metallic taste in the mouth. They can get mouth ulcers (aphthae), various problems with the teeth, and copious sweating day and night that doesn't bring relief. When they have throat and mouth problems, the tongue swells up, so that the imprints of the teeth are visible. The ear-nose-throat (ENT) area is very sensitive in *Mercurius* children. Inflammation often occurs in the throat and ear, sometimes with discharges of pus and blood. We also see muscle twitches, stuttering, or a quivering voice.

The gut is also a sensitive organ in *Mercurius* children. They can get diarrhea with gut cramps, also illnesses such as ulcerative colitis (chronic inflammation of the large intestine) or Crohn's disease (chronic inflammation of the gastrointestinal tract).

Many complaints get worse at night.

Food and Drink

It's noticeable that they either have a strong desire for butter (also bread and butter) or a strong dislike of it. They love sweet things and cold drinks and often have an aversion to meat.

The Natrium carbonicum Child

Sodium carbonate, Washing soda, Soda ash (Na_2CO_3)

Mineral remedy

"Careful with relationships"

Origin

The remedy *Natrium carbonicum* is made from sodium carbonate. Hahnemann described in his "Materia Medica Pura" exactly how this remedy is made. This salt consists of two elements, sodium and carbon. Our knowledge of these two chemical elements has enabled us to reach a deeper understanding of the remedy picture of *Natrium carbonicum*.

Sodium fits the stage of life when the child begins to form relationships with other people. The first relationship is obviously with the mother. This is why *Natrium muriaticum* is one of the most frequently prescribed remedies. The next relationship — when the child develops normally — is with the father figure. The remedy *Natrium carbonicum* fits this.

Carbon symbolically represents the father and everything that symbolizes the father, especially the concept of "self-worth." See also the remedy picture of *Graphites*.

Gentle and reserved

Natrium carbonicum children are sensitive children who appear somewhat shy. They're very sensitive to moods, like *Phosphorus* children, but less open. In relationships, they're very cautious. Since they're very vulnerable, they don't open up easily. There's mostly a reason in their lives for this reserve, since they're basically spontaneous and sociable. At some time, they noticed that not everyone has the same delicacy as they do, which shocked them. They react especially sensitively to how people treat them - or rather, whether people respect them as they are. If their parents or other children offend them, they tend to retreat. They aren't fighters and don't have much aggression in them. They're masters at appearing on the

175

outside to be mild and compliant while feeling very sad and lonely on the inside.

Problems with the father figure

As already mentioned, their main problem is with the father figure in their lives. This can be the father himself or it might also be a teacher or a sports coach.

The hurt lying deepest inside the *Natrium carbonicum* child is rejection by the father. Every child has the need for a good relationship with their father. If the father, however, doesn't accept the child, the *Natrium carbonicum* child shuts him- or herself off. In this way, these children try to protect their self-worth and to avoid being hurt again. The same pattern can also arise when the father is absent for other reasons, for example, due to separation or death. Inside, the children feel rejected. Since they can't rationalize these experiences, they put themselves at the center of events and so experience the loss as a personal debasement: "He's gone because he finds me worthless."

Deep inside, they know that it's not really like that, that they are indeed worthy, but they'll do anything to avoid being hurt again in that way. They protect their dignity by withdrawing.

Special instinct

Natrium carbonicum children possess a special instinct for the mood and temperament of other people. Without having spoken with a person, they mostly know very well what the other person is like. They immediately feel sympathy or dislike and these feelings are seldom wrong. If they don't like someone, they won't show it. They can be very friendly to this person, yet inside they feel dislike, which can express itself in various physical reactions.

Their sensitivity often causes them to feel unwell when there's a change in air pressure, and they can sense a storm or a thunderstorm in advance. A sensitivity to music, especially piano music, is characteristic of *Natrium carbonicum* children. This can be so pronounced that they just can't tolerate piano music. *Graphites* children have the same sensitivity to organ music!

This oversensitivity is the origin of allergic reactions to many different things, especially to food.

Excluded

Natrium carbonicum children find it difficult to establish contact with the outside world. They quickly feel excluded and have the feeling of being shut out, as if there was something separating them from other people, which prevents them establishing a connection. If the outside world reacts in a hostile manner, this is another confirmation of their "expulsion." Sadly, *Natrium carbonicum* children can arouse negative reactions in others by their reserved and withdrawn behavior, which makes them all too often the victim.

Natrium carbonicum can help these children to achieve more of a feeling of self-worth and self-confidence, to open up more to the outside world. This helps them to respect themselves more, which means they automatically earn more respect from others!

Physical symptoms

The same emotional issues are reflected in the stomach and gut complaints. The more they repress their feelings, the more their stomach goes wild. The more sensitively they react to moods, the more strongly they react to food. Allergies often occur in *Natrium carbonicum* children.

In general, they feel the cold and are sensitive to drafts. They also tolerate the sun poorly, as it gives them headaches. *Natrium carbonicum* is one of the most important remedies for sunstroke.

Their weak ankles can be seen as symbolic for their lack of (fatherly) support, which prevents them from standing on their own two feet and purposefully entering the outside world.

Food and Drink

The most obvious thing is their dislike of milk and their bad reaction to it. Every drop can irritate their gut and lead to diarrhea.

The Natrium muriaticum Child

Common salt, Sodium chloride (NaCl)

Mineral remedy

"A protective wall"

Origin

We think of common salt as a simple substance that's not particularly valuable. This is due to the fact that, for us, salt is present in abundance. But for the people of Tibet or the Sahara, for example, salt is one of the most valuable things there is. A human being can't survive long without salt!

Sodium and chloride are very important in our bodies, just like calcium, iron, potassium, phosphorus, and many more. Too much or too little of these substances leads to major physical illness. Therefore, our bodies have amazing mechanisms to very precisely regulate the concentrations of these minerals.

A new way of looking at this commonly used remedy is to think of it in terms of its two constituent elements, sodium and chloride. Both sodium and chloride are concerned with interpersonal relations. Sodium stands for whether or not to enter a relationship, while chloride stands for the loss of a relationship, specifically the connection with the mother.

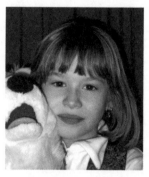
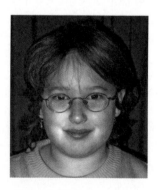

Nat-m.   *Nat-m.*

Going without or losing care

The first bond that a child makes after birth is with the mother. She is generally the source of care and attention. In modern psychology, it's become very clear that going without a mother figure causes many problems that — if not sufficiently treated — can affect a person's whole life right into old age. The mother provides the young child with the basis for future development.

Natrium muriaticum as a homeopathic remedy is able, even many years later, to help people overcome the wounds caused by the lack or loss of the mother figure.

Situations in which the *Natrium muriaticum* picture can arise include a period in an incubator, the death of the mother, or some other kind of separation from the mother as a very young child. In many cases in which a *Natrium muriaticum* picture arises, it's not so much the physical absence of the mother as the fact that she herself has problems giving attention and genuine care.

Reserved

Natrium muriaticum children are mostly reserved, not because they're anxious like *Calcarea carbonica*, but because they feel so vulnerable. They only allow people they trust completely to gain access to their inner world. They're very sensitive children who often care for other people. Yet when they themselves are missing something, they first want to be left in peace before possibly speaking about it later on. Be sure to allow them this time! They would certainly like a warm relationship, but they're afraid of being hurt, especially when they've already had a bad experience. One hint for this can be that they avoid eye contact. This is, however, nothing to do with dishonesty, but is rather to do with these children's oversensitivity. By looking someone in the eye, you enter into that person's world, and this is something the *Natrium muriaticum* child will only permit someone they completely trust!

All-or-nothing relationships

Natrium muriaticum children are very sensitive and, therefore, also very vulnerable. Just like *Natrium carbonicum* children, they're mostly musical and are very moved by beautiful music. Externally, they

179

appear to be strong and independent, like a child who doesn't really need other people.

On the inside, they can feel lonely and abandoned. If they allow someone into their world, it's for ever. In friendships and relationships, it's "everything or nothing" for them. They usually only have a few friends, but will go through hell and high water for them! Salt serves to protect fish from going bad, which exactly reflects how *Natrium muriaticum* children do everything to preserve their friendships.

Safekeeping

Since they can listen very well, are very sensitive, and are excellent at keeping secrets — they know from their own experience how painful it is if secrets are passed on — other children often turn to them to tell their problems. It's really striking how others are always confiding their cares and problems in them. Other children feel that they're good listeners who won't condemn straightaway. Everyone needs such people to listen to them. *Natrium muriaticum* children take others seriously. They regard what's told them in confidence as a personal secret.

Wall

"Muriaticum" contains the word "muur" (Dutch for wall). To protect themselves from the tough outer world, *Natrium muriaticum* children sometimes build a protective wall around themselves, even when very young. This shield, however, doesn't just keep out the outside world. It also causes emotions to be blocked. Fury and annoyance can affect them internally without often being expressed. To show emotions is still seen as a sign of weakness in our society, whereas someone who puts on a brave face is seen as strong. *Natrium muriaticum* children carry this message deep inside, because they've often picked up this pattern from home.

Of course, such a pattern can also arise later in life, for example, due to an emotional injury. "That will never happen to me again!" is the reaction, and the door is slammed shut. Emotions are then no longer expressed — often for years on end. It requires a lot of confidence before *Natrium muriaticum* children will once again speak of their worries. When they're given *Natrium muriaticum*, they realize that the best solution is to talk and express things.

Physical symptoms

To dissolve salt, moisture is necessary. This is why *Natrium muriaticum* children often have a disturbance in the way their bodies deal with moisture. On the one hand, the skin and mucous membranes are often dry, whereas on the other hand, they tend to retain moisture so that edemas occur. Headaches due to unexpressed emotions, staying in the sun, or — in older girls — before menstruation are typical of this remedy. A further example of the "holding on" is constipation, which is worsened by dryness in the gut.

Natrium muriaticum children like somewhat cooler weather and love being in the open. At the seaside, they feel better (in exceptional cases, they can feel worse), since they have more space there. For this reason, they avoid small and oppressive rooms.

Many *Natrium muriaticum* children have fever blisters or other fluid-filled small blisters. They frequently have a crack in the middle of the lower lip. "Geographic tongue" (mapped tongue) is also characteristic of this remedy.

Food and Drink

Not surprisingly, they have a desire for salt and are very thirsty. The relationship to the sea is expressed in the desire for fish. In addition, they like bread, pasta, and bitter things. Fat disgusts them and they also tolerate it poorly.

Natrium muriaticum in the Clinic

Maartje's difficulties with writing

Ten-year-old Maartje came for her learning difficulties. Especially when writing, she made many mistakes. She twisted words and sometimes wrote as if in a mirror, but generally she could read well. She had a motor weakness and had problems keeping up in gymnastics. Her clumsiness often attracted attention. Moreover, she got a headache before it began to snow, coughed a lot, and often had a cold. At school she was often teased.

Due to her low birth weight, Maartje was kept in an incubator for a day before she had contact with her mother. A few weeks after her birth, her maternal grandmother died unexpectedly.

She was a calm, careful child. "She first checks which way the wind's blowing," her mother explained to me, "and she prefers being alone to playing with other children." Maartje was guided by emotion, couldn't stand harsh words, loved music, and was crazy about animals. When she was in pain or was worried about something, she just wanted to be left alone. But when other children had problems, she was always eager to help them. Then she was very loving and caring. Due to the problems at school, she had low self-confidence.

The problems mentioned above (difficulties writing, clumsiness, as well as the physical symptoms) fit the picture of *Natrium muriaticum* well, as does her character (tendency to withdraw, especially when worried, empathetic, and reserved). At the time I prescribed the remedy, it wasn't known that *Natrium muriaticum* is good for children who've been in an incubator, or better still, for children who've lost contact with the mother at an important stage in their lives. The loss of someone, in this case the grandmother, can similarly bring forth a *Natrium muriaticum* picture.

Therefore, it's not surprising that Maartje reacted sensationally to *Natrium muriaticum*. On the second day after taking it, she spontaneously cried, and since then she continuously improved. She felt emotionally better, no longer had headaches, could write more easily, and was no longer teased. Her motor development remained weak, for which she had some additional therapy. It was only necessary to repeat the remedy one year later.

182

The Nux vomica Child

Poison nut, Strychnine tree, Quaker buttons

Plant remedy (Loganiaceae family)

"Ambitious"

Origin

Nux vomica is made from the seeds of the fruit of the strychnine tree, which grows in north Australia, in Sri Lanka, and elsewhere. In Hahnemann's time, the seeds were often used medicinally, and so he decided to conduct a remedy proving with them. It became one of his most frequently prescribed remedies, well-suited to modern times — to "stressed-out" modern people! In the meantime, the remedy picture has become clearer, and we now know very well what kind of child corresponds to this remedy.

The seeds of this fruit contain copper (also known as a homeopathic remedy, *Cuprum metallicum* — see the chapter in this book), which explains a lot about the picture of *Nux vomica*. Copper leads to cramps and suits a certain kind of obsessive restlessness.

In herbal medicine too, poison nut has been used as long as anyone can remember. For example, in India the bitter-tasting bark of the tree is administered for fever (including malaria) and snakebites. An infusion of the leaves is used for rheumatic complaints.

The poison nut belongs to the Loganiaceae family. The German name *"Brechnuss"* ("vomiting nut") gives an indication of the effect, since the seeds contain substances that induce stomach cramps and nausea.

Determined and independent

Nux vomica children have a strong personality. They know very well what they want and like to hold on to the reins. They're little "managers in the making." Even as newborn babies, they love peace and quiet. They like to be alone and can take care of themselves well.

As long as they're dependent on others, they want their wishes to be fulfilled as quickly as possible. As newborns, they need to eat

183

straightaway when they're hungry. If they're in the playpen and they see something that they want to play with, they insist on it being given to them immediately. As soon as they're able to, they do things on their own. They don't like being dependent on other people and, in any case, they think they can do everything better.

Passionate and ambitious

In everything they do, they give their best. They're ambitious, and – even when very young – they want to be the best at everything. They don't make it easy for themselves, yet they're also critical of others. Everything has to happen at full steam and in no time. When they're trying hard to do something, they give 200% effort, as if they're constantly trying to prove themselves to the outside world. Their passion and ambition grow accordingly if they're weak in a particular area. For example, if they're smaller than their peers, they'll have an even bigger need to perform exceptionally well in some other area. We often see this theme in remedies from the Loganiaceae family, which also includes *Ignatia*, *Gelsemium*, and *Spigelia*. Yet *Nux vomica* children show the greatest passion.

Aiming high

In many respects, these children resemble *Aurum* children. They have the same ambition, passion, sincerity, and a strong sense of responsibility. But *Nux vomica* children are less complicated and mostly more optimistic by nature. Impatience and restlessness are qualities they share with *Aurum* children. Once they're busy with something, they find it very difficult to stop. They don't allow themselves any rest, although they sometimes really need it. Problems are there to be solved for these children, and they certainly don't go out of their way to avoid them. No, they tend to actually seek out difficult challenges. They need instead to be encouraged to take a break now and again and to lower their sights!

Flare up quickly

The downside is that they have a considerable amount of aggression, which they don't try to hide! Even when they're playing sport, they always give it 100%. In team games, they're not always pleasant to play with. Fellow players who aren't trying hard enough often get their comeuppance, as *Nux vomica* children aren't particularly tolerant. They expect others — exactly as they expect themselves — to give everything. And if the game is lost, it's best to leave them in peace!

When they're overloaded with homework over a long period or when they're suffering from "leisure stress" — which is nowadays unfortunately all too common — they can become very irritable, and they can flare up when someone disturbs them. Yet they don't hold on to their anger for long, since they're unable to do so. When circumstances don't allow them to express their rage, they get physical complaints such as headaches and stomach cramps.

Considerate

Even if *Nux vomica* children can get into a proper rage and show little patience, they're also very considerate of their fellow human beings. They're possibly not as sympathetic as *Phosphorus* or *Causticum* children and don't like "softies" (children who are too sensitive), yet they also don't like it when something unjust happens to another child. They love sincerity and openness. They themselves are open and sincere, and they expect that from other people too. Their way of helping is above all practical.

Their sensitivity is particularly pronounced when it comes to music. If a piece of music touches them, they can even cry. Other impressions also affect them deeply. They're very sensitive to noise and smell. They don't miss anything. They notice when something hasn't been done correctly, such as a picture that's not hanging straight. Exactly like *Arsenicum album* children, they're perfectionists as far as external appearance goes, not so much from fear (as in *Arsenicum*) as out of a striving for perfection.

Being busy

Nux vomica children become unsettled if they have to sit still, and therefore don't like going on visits with their family. They have more important things to do. They feel that they're worth something when they're achieving things. That can come partly from their upbringing, but it also comes from their own character. A

185

challenge is what they like best of all. Straightforward routine tasks quickly bore them. They're always looking for something to push up against, something to fight for or defend themselves against. Things must always go as they wish, since they can't tolerate contradiction. This characteristic gives them a charismatic touch, but it's also their pitfall. There's a danger that they ignore their own limits and so don't get enough relaxation. They become exhausted, sleep poorly – particularly at 3 a.m. they can lie awake for hours – and become irritable. That they might be difficult doesn't even occur to them, yet for the other family members they can be impossible. We often hear the parents saying how, after a dose of *Nux vomica*, the house is once again at peace.

Physical symptoms

The complaints that we particularly see in *Nux vomica* babies and small children are colds as well as left-sided umbilical or inguinal hernias. In newborn babies, colds can cause serious breathing difficulties if they don't automatically switch to breathing through the mouth. *Nux vomica* is one of the most important remedies for this.

Under normal circumstances, *Nux vomica* children are not so liable to get ill, as they generally have a pretty robust constitution. Only drafts and cold can weaken them, causing colds or muscle complaints (in the neck and back). They like warmth and they can easily tolerate even great heat. Many complaints are noticeably improved by warmth.

Their nervous system is the most sensitive to illness. If they take on too much or can't cope with worries or tension, serious illness can develop. Then especially the gastrointestinal tract goes crazy. They get cramps, acidic burping, vomiting, and even stomach inflammation, as well as difficulty passing their stool, accompanied by a sensitive and distended abdomen.

Similar to *Cuprum* children, who also get ill from too much inner tension, *Nux vomica* children easily get muscle cramps, especially in the neck and back, which can lead to headaches or even migraines. A single dose of this remedy helps them to unwind better and to view things in a more relaxed way.

186

Food and Drink

Nux vomica children love seasoned, fat, and bitter foods. There are only a few things that they don't like, but they need to watch out with the amounts. It's better if they avoid alcohol and coffee when they get older. They need these things to get rid of their tension, but they're precisely what cause them problems!

Nux vomica in the Clinic

Sickly child

Jost was a little rascal. At fourteen months, he was already "all there." Everything he saw, he wanted to examine closely, and he reacted irritably when he wasn't able to or wasn't allowed to.

His mother brought him to see me because he had been sickly for months. Jost often had a cold, which mostly turned into rasping breathing, ending up as bronchitis. Apart from this, he was very irritable, hardly wanted to eat, and slept poorly. Recently, he had been regularly waking up between 03:30 and 04:00 (3:30 and 4 a.m.).

As far as eating was concerned, he was quickly full and didn't like warm food. He loved acidic food like grapefruit. After eating, his abdomen swelled up. Jost easily got cold.

He went to a kindergarten where he had great fun. Jost had a strong will and was afraid of nothing. When he did something that he wasn't allowed to do, he was very difficult to correct, since punishment hardly affected him. He was constantly aware of everything going on around him, and it was noticeable how quickly he was able to see the connections between things.

His family history included tuberculosis and asthma. His mother was also prone to colds.

After a dose of *Nux vomica*, the change began to take hold. Jost became more cheerful and full of the joys of life. After a week, he felt better and the colds disappeared. He still didn't eat warm food, but he frequently grabbed a piece of bread or fruit. Unlike before, he now began to gain weight and soon reached the appropriate weight for his age.

After 6 months — in the middle of winter — he had a setback. He got a cold and I recommended another dose of *Nux vomica*. There was no improvement. In view of the family history, I decided to give him a dose of *Tuberculinum*, following which his cold disappeared.

After another 6 months, I saw Jost again. His mood was as it had been a year ago, and also the physical complaints - colds with coughing and rasping breath — had started again. *Tuberculinum* brought no improvement, but after a dose of *Nux vomica* his overall state of health improved as well as his mood. Since then he's had two more doses of *Nux vomica* in the space of a year.

The Opium Child

Opium poppy, Papaver somniferum

Plant remedy (Papaveraceae family)

"Numb with shock"

Origin

Opium is the most important product of the opium poppy (*Papaver somniferum*). Since time immemorial, this plant has been highly valued by healers. In ancient China, opium was written about thousands of years ago, both for its healing powers and for the problems that can arise when it's used improperly.

Opium contains various alkaloids, of which the best known are morphine and codeine. There's probably no medicine on earth that's used and abused more often. It's not only a strong painkiller; it also helps people to forget their emotional pain. The pleasurable state in which people find themselves after taking it is the most important reason for dependency on opium and its derivatives, of which heroin is the most notorious. Morphine is also used as a painkiller and codeine as a cough remedy.

Hahnemann himself introduced *Opium* as a homeopathic remedy. In his introduction to this remedy, he stresses that homeopathic "*Opium*" is intended to support the process of healing, not to be used as a painkiller. It can obviously have the effect of reducing pain, but only after the source of the pain has been removed.

In (small) children it can be an important remedy. Not particularly because it fits a particular type of child, but because it can resolve the negative consequences caused by shock and fear in the mother during pregnancy and birth.

Shock and deadening

An *Opium* picture can be triggered by an intense shock in children. This often arises from the fear experienced by the mother during pregnancy or birth, which the child picks up. It's known from psychological studies that even children in the womb are vulnerable to

189

the emotions of the mother. Obviously, the fright or the shock can occur later, in a newborn baby or in an older child. Nevertheless, the *Opium* picture can also be caused by other emotions such as shame. It can also arise when the mother received a strong painkiller or an anesthetic, which unfortunately leaves traces in the child.

Sleepy or agile

Children showing an *Opium* picture can be either sleepy or very agile. In the first case, they sleep a lot and deeply, and are hard to wake. In the second case, they're wide awake and find it hard to fall asleep. Apart from this, they take fright at the slightest noise. Their sense of hearing is acute and they're aware of everything.

An intermediate form is the "waking coma." The children appear to be awake yet in reality nothing gets through to them. The deadened state can go so far that the children react to nothing anymore. They appear to be isolated in their own world, as we can also see with autistic children.

The sleepy children cause the most concern, as they're often lethargic and slow in whatever they do. When asleep, they breathe deeply and snore, and the breathing can stop from time to time. Obviously other measures are necessary here, such as a special device to wake the parents when the child hasn't breathed for a long period.

Oblivious to pain

A further striking symptom shown by *Opium* is the reduced or absent sense of pain in children. The nerve impulses are not conducted or only with a delay. This is a neurological problem. Yet even on the emotional level, these children can be "deadened." If something awful happens, they don't feel it and express themselves accordingly: "Everything's fine!" — even when the situation is very serious and painful. The cause can be physical pain as well as psychological trauma, such as violence in war or incest. In this case, the deadening is a natural defense mechanism to protect against the intolerable pain.

In such situations, our body releases substances called endorphins, which are very similar to opium. In this state, children can feel very happy and can just dream away. They're like people who have smoked opium and drifted into a dreamy rapture. But if children get stuck in this deadened state, they need help, as the deadening not only dulls their pain but also prevents healing of the underlying trauma. In addition, along with a suitable homeopathic remedy, the help of a professional psychologist is necessary here!

Fear and fits of rage

As we can observe with many remedy pictures, *Opium* shows two contrary reaction patterns. Along with the deadening and the dreaminess, we also see enormous fears and sudden, extreme fits of rage.

The fears are mostly the consequence of an earlier shock. Since the cause is often only found in the unconscious, the fears appear to have no connection to anything. Children can be afraid of everything imaginable, and they sometimes have dreadful visions. The perceptions of other sense organs can also evoke threatening feelings, such as a foreign smell or taste that has no connection to current reality. Older children often express their fear as "fear of fear." It can be an overpowering feeling for them.

Fear is an important cause of the fits of rage, which is similar to what we can very easily see in animals – the worst aggression arises out of fear. In their rage and annoyance, these children redden and their pupils either contract or expand. Such a fit of rage can be very frightening, because the child loses all control and then behaves very rashly.

Physical symptoms

Along with the sleepiness, lethargy, and the diminished sense of pain, the sensitivity to warmth is possibly the most noticeable symptom. *Opium* children can't tolerate warmth. In bed, they seek the coolest spot to sleep. Due to their inner heat, they sweat easily, on the head as well as the rest of the body.

On the neurological level, many different symptoms are possible, such as trembling, involuntary shaking, epileptic fits, or – on the contrary – an almost comatose state.

Opium is an important homeopathic remedy for children who frequently suffer from persistent constipation or hard, round stools.

The bowels are so lethargic that they seem to be paralyzed. Even if the constipation started after an anesthetic, *Opium* can help.

Sleep is either very deep or very superficial with snoring. Their sleep is disturbed by nightmares and terrifying images of monstrous creatures, dark figures, and similar things.

The remedy *Opium* is invaluable in healing the deep causes of all these problems.

The Phosphorus Child

Phosphorus (P). Mineral remedy

"Looking for contact"

Origin

For weakened *Phosphorus* types, Hahnemann recommends — as well as giving them the homeopathic remedy — having a well-meaning, strong, and healthy person hold the hands of the patient or lay their hands on the weakened part of the patient's body for several minutes. This is now known as "therapeutic touch," the affectionate touch used by nursing staff in hospital. And people needing *Phosphorus*, especially children, are indeed sensitive to touch.

The chemical element phosphorus was discovered in the year 1669, and got its name "phosphorus" (Greek for "carrier of light") from its phosphorescent (light-emitting) quality. Phosphorus catches fire easily, and is therefore used to make matches.

In plants, animals, and the human body, phosphorus is an essential substance. *Phosphorus* compounds are used in the basic construction and function of organisms, such as in the energy supply. Disturbances in phosphorus metabolism primarily affect the nervous system. There's a Dutch saying that shows the importance of phos-

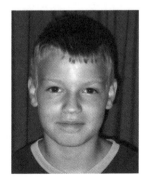

Phos.

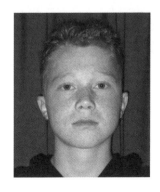

Phos.

193

phorus for concentration: "Without phosphorus, there would be no thoughts."

Communicative

Phosphorus children are extremely sociable. Due to their need for contact, they love company. When the mood is good, they're like fish in water. At school, they form friendships easily and are open to everyone. They hate being alone since they need contact to feel safe and secure. The presence of other people gives them a feeling of protection and warmth. If someone is not feeling well, they sense it immediately — so strongly do they feel connected with other people. They can't tolerate it when someone else is feeling unwell, and they want to help them straightaway. They themselves suffer when someone else is suffering.

Friendly contact

Phosphorus children are particularly looking for contact with friends. Friends — this can include siblings — are more important than anything else. The loss of a friendship – for example, due to a move – is hard for them to come to terms with. Material things concern them less. It's always about people.

They're very sensitive to the prevailing mood, and many children are so open that they possess clairvoyant qualities. This sensitivity can also make them nervous and fearful, especially when it's dark or before a storm or a thunderstorm. In the dark, where they can't see other people, they feel alone. The fear of ghosts plays a role here, not only due to their sensitivity but also due to their strong fantasy. Although they don't like arguments, they can easily get furious. *Phosphorus* is easily inflammable! But usually this anger is quickly over. They aren't children who hold grudges. Most of all, they just want to be good friends again.

Carriers of light

These children have an intense radiance. Their eyes and hair can shine. Due to their brightness, they automatically become the center of attention, although they don't consciously bring this about. It's not so much about the need for attention as in *Pulsatilla* children, or for recognition and respect as in *Aurum* children, but rather the need to feel connected with other people.

Phosphorus children can communicate well. They learn languages playfully, they like holding conversations and mostly writing too. Since communication doesn't just function at the level of words, *Phosphorus* children also love physical contact, since this enables them to share something of their own love. They also receive energy from others through touch. Hahnemann already described this in his introduction to this remedy. Many complaints can be improved by massage or touch. It's not so much something like the kneading of muscles as the exchange of energy. Light touch is enough for this.

Learning and helping

Along with conscientiously keeping up with old contacts — good friends are for a lifetime — they like to form new friendships. Even when very young, they like getting to know new people and investigating new areas of interest. Their social and intellectual interests are wide-ranging. They love going out and traveling, since this lets them satisfy their curiosity, and they can learn about something new.

Everyone comes across problems in their life, and suffering is unavoidable. We can help one another to solve problems or to come to terms with them, but we aren't in a position to take over other people's problems. For *Phosphorus* children, it's very hard to accept this, yet they still tend to try doing it. This causes them to suffer too instead of just showing sympathy. The difference is subtle, but very important for their health, since they lose energy to others in this way - energy that they need themselves to stay on an even keel. The person who receives the energy may well be glad, but they must realize that they have to solve their own problems in the end.

The homeopathic remedy *Phosphorus* can help *Phosphorus* children to maintain their boundaries and to make sure that their energy is used in a sensible way.

Physical symptoms

In many books, *Phosphorus* children are described in terms of their external features. Our experience is that this is certainly helpful in recognizing the picture, but it can never be decisive. *Phosphorus* children can just as well be small and plump as tall and slender. Luckily, there are a number of physical symptoms that are typical for *Phosphorus* people.

We often see an increased tendency to bleed. Small wounds continue bleeding for a long time – for example, after a tooth has been extracted. They quickly get bruised and suffer subcutaneous bleeding. Nose bleeds are more common than in other types.

Phosphorus and *Sulfur* are the remedies best suited to burning pains. These pains can occur anywhere in the body, especially in the stomach. The pain is relieved in the short term by drinking or eating something cold, but as soon as the stomach contents have warmed up, the burning starts again.

Most of the pains that *Phosphorus* children have are relieved by massage or touch, since they react very well to the affection and warmth of other people.

Phosphorus can cover illnesses of the respiratory tract very well, such as bronchitis or lung inflammation, and it also helps hoarseness and problems of concentration. Too much studying can mentally exhaust *Phosphorus* children.

One characteristic that we often see in *Phosphorus* is that they can only sleep on the right side. They'll never sleep on the left side!

Food and Drink

Phosphorus children love cold drinks, milk shakes, and ice cream and are often crazy about chocolate. They either like or dislike fish and sweet things.

Phosphorus in the Clinic

Paula: allergy, eczema, and headache

Paula had had skin problems since she was a baby. A major bout of eczema had healed on its own, but when she came to me — she was now nine years old — she was suffering from stubborn eczema between the toes. Her eyes also itched when she was riding. The most important symptom at this time was her headaches. She had these when she had slept too little due to tension, sometimes of a positive kind as at Christmas or on her birthday, but also due to negative emotions. When she had slept well, the headaches improved again.

Various allergies and also asthma ran in her family. In the previous generation, some of the family members had undergone a course of treatment for tuberculosis.

She was a gentle, simple, and open child. Her mother said she was very fearful when she was alone or in the dark. She had to have the light on in her room. She loved people and animals. Horses were her favorite animals.

She loved fish. She didn't like cheese so much. She always slept on her right side.

After a dose of *Phosphorus*, her state of health improved so much — she no longer had headaches, the itching stopped, and the eczema disappeared — that we decided to only see her again if her complaints returned.

The Pulsatilla Child

Small pasque flower, Windflower, Anemone pratensis (anemos = wind;
pulsare = move)

Plant remedy (Ranunculaceae family)

"Need for comfort"

Origin

Pulsatilla is one of the most outstanding homeopathic remedies, since it corresponds to an "archetypal" human type. According to many homeopaths, the picture of *Pulsatilla* stands for Eve, the first woman. As a medicine, it definitely relates to motherhood and to becoming a mother. It's always been used for women who are involuntarily childless but otherwise in good health. And many of them become pregnant.

When we take a look at this sweet – in the true sense of the word – plant, we can learn much about the character of the child who needs it.

"Anemos" means literally "breath" or "wind" and "pulsare" means "move." In England, this anemone is not for nothing called "windflower." This plant dances at the slightest breath of wind.

Still more impressive is the sentence uttered by the famous herbalist Dodanaeus about *Pulsatilla*: "The flower called anemone grew from

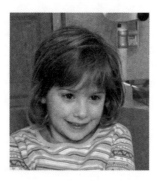

Puls.

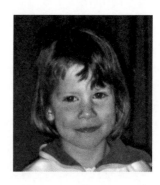

Puls.

the tears wept on the earth by Venus as she mourned her young Adonis."
Pulsatilla grows especially in sunny areas on sandy earth. The plant contains much silica, which is why it has many similarities with the remedy *Silicea* (silicon dioxide).

Tender and likeable

Pulsatilla children usually have a likeable and gentle character. They may be a bit shy to start with, but as soon as they get to know someone, they come out of themselves. They love company and really blossom when they notice that others like them. They need attention and have a desire for tender loving care. It seems to be a remedy that only fits girls, yet in practice it's regularly and success-fully used also for boys. These boys are mostly sensitive and mild. They also like tender loving care and it's not out of the ordinary for a thirteen-year-old *Pulsatilla* boy to jump onto his mother's lap for a cuddle!
Just as the flower bends to the wind, so do *Pulsatilla* children adapt to the people around them. They know how pleasant it is when people are likeable and friendly. All plants of the Ranunculaceae family, including also *Staphisagria* and *Aconitum*, want people to get on with each other in a respectful way. They find it hard to put up with injustice and rudeness. *Pulsatilla* children only feel good when they know that they're loved. When they feel well, they themselves can give much love.

Motherly

Pulsatilla girls are little "mommies" from an early age. They play with dolls and love caring for other children as if these were babies. Yet they themselves also like playing the baby. They're familiar with this role. They sense very well what others want, and will do everything they can to try and fulfill these wishes.
In view of this caring attitude, it's reasonable to suppose that even very young *Pulsatilla* girls have the desire to be a mother. *Pulsatilla* corresponds to the goddess Venus, or Aphrodite in Greek, which is the symbol of the original mother, like Mary in the Christian world. Due to their need for warmth and care, they love friendly get-

199

togethers. "Cozy" is a word they like to use. In good company, they feel like a fish in water, assuming they get the necessary attention. After all, the driving force behind their life is attention and loving care, without which they waste away.

Emotional and in need of comfort

The feelings of *Pulsatilla* children can fluctuate wildly. One moment, they're deeply miserable, then a second later they can be beaming happily again. Their life is determined by their emotions and there's nothing they can do about it. That's where their strength and their vulnerability both lie.

For girls in puberty, who have already started to menstruate, this comes out very strongly. In the days before menstruation, they have severe mood swings. Without any obvious reason, they can suddenly start crying. For other people, especially their friends, this is very hard to understand. "You can't just cry like that, can you?" They certainly can. *Pulsatilla* girls sometimes just want to weep. In particular, they can be overcome by a feeling of loneliness. This feeling can be so strong that they feel as if they're completely alone in the world. To drive out the loneliness, they look for warmth and comfort. Then they're also very happy when their father, their mother, or a nice friend is around to console them!

Pulsatilla obviously can't transform these children. They remain emotional, and indeed there's nothing wrong with that. But the remedy helps them to develop a more stable emotional balance, so that they're not bowled over by every passing "breath of wind." If *Pulsatilla* fits well, it's also able to heal the physical complaints.

Physical symptoms

Before *Pulsatilla* was used as a homeopathic remedy, the plant had been used for eye complaints, especially for inflammations with a mild, yellow discharge. *Pulsatilla* children also have the same discharge when they have a cold, which frequently turns into an ear infection.

Whatever complaints *Pulsatilla* children have, from eczema to joint complaints, fresh air always does them good. They don't like small rooms at all. When they play in the open, they often get well by themselves, especially when there's a fresh wind blowing. That's why they love the beach, as long as it's not too hot.

Pulsatilla is one of the remedies strongly related to female hormones. *Pulsatilla* girls often have complaints to do with menstruation. Beforehand, they usually feel even more emotionally labile than normal and often suffer from abdominal pains and headaches. Just as their feelings are changeable, so their menstrual bleeding can vary in duration and intensity. Sometimes their periods can disappear for months at a time, before returning at very short intervals.

Yet for all complaints it's true that comfort brings relief.

Food and Drink

In the same way that they like fresh weather, *Pulsatilla* children also like fresh food. Raw fruit and vegetables and light food suits them best, whereas they can't tolerate heavy and fatty food well. Fatty food quickly makes them feel sick. It's noticeable that they don't have much thirst. They really have to take care to drink the necessary amount of fluid each day.

Pulsatilla in the Clinic

Vera and her sensitive bowels

Vera was one year old when her mother brought her to see me. From the time when her mother ceased to breastfeed her, at around the age of 7 months, she had been getting red skin rashes. She reacted to various foods, such as milk products, eggs, oranges, and nectarines. Her gut was also very sensitive and reacted to the same foods. She quickly got cold hands, but in general she was always warm. She preferred to be outside and her complaints improved in the fresh air.

Vera was very likeable and open. She had blond hair and blue eyes, was pleasant, happy, and laughed a lot. She loved company and liked going out. The more friends she had, the better she felt. She wasn't afraid of strangers and had very few fears. She just didn't like small rooms, and she was frightened by loud noises.

After a dose of *Pulsatilla*, her health was much better. In the following months, she needed another dose of *Pulsatilla* now and again.

Sandra's ear infections

In her short life — she wasn't even one year old yet — Sandra had already had four ear infections. She was five months old when she caught her first cold. From that time on, her hearing seemed to be affected too. The ear infections had all been treated with antibiotics. She slept well and had a healthy appetite. She loved fruit, bread, and milk. In bed and when she was drinking, she sweated heavily on her head.

Sandra was very likeable, lively, and happy. She already had a will of her own and liked to have lots of people around her. She enjoyed the coziness, liking to sit on people's laps and cuddle up to them. When she was sad, she liked to be comforted.

After a dose of *Pulsatilla*, Sandra quickly felt better. The colds disappeared and her hearing improved.

In the following two years, she needed a dose of *Pulsatilla* every six months to stop colds developing. When I saw her again five years later, everything had been going well. But she had recently had ear problems again, and obviously I prescribed *Pulsatilla* once more.

The Saccharum officinale Child

Sugar cane

Plant remedy

"Soothing sugar"

Origin

My first experience with fresh sugar cane was in the Dominican Republic. After a walk in the tropical forest lasting several hours, we came to a settlement. Our tour guide asked a woman for a piece of sugar cane that was lying in her garden. Smiling broadly, she cut us each a huge piece and waited for our reaction to the taste. It tasted as cool as ice cream, as sweet as honey, fantastic, nutritious, and at the same time thirst-quenching. Exactly what we needed after such a hike! There was simply no comparison with the sugar that's manufactured from it. Our grinning faces spoke for themselves and, without asking, she cut us each another piece.

A remedy for our times

Sugar consumption has increased massively compared to earlier times. This is despite warnings from dieticians and dentists about excessive consumption. The influential homeopath Constantin Hering made it clear 150 years ago that sugar could cause many illnesses. Apparently we need more sugar than our ancestors. But why? What does sugar mean?

Sugar is love; the term "sugar" is, after all, a term of endearment! Children who need the remedy *Saccharum* yearn for attention, love, and affection, and will do anything to get this. They're often crazy about sugar, which seems to have a soothing effect when they're restless. It seems as if *Saccharum* is one of the most important remedies for agitated children. The *Saccharum* picture often occurs in adults, but in children it's easier to recognize. It's probably true that *Saccharum* is simply more often indicated in children.

Fear of being abandoned

Behind the strong desire for love and attention, *Saccharum* children feel a lack of self-love. For this reason, they're afraid to lose the mother's love, and therefore they demand it completely. They're very afraid of being abandoned. In addition, at night they like most of all to sleep in bed with their mother.

The reason is often that there is indeed a lack of attention, and at the same time a considerable and natural need for attention. Different factors can play a role here, including actual neglect, but also a lack of bodily contact. This is why breast-feeding is so important for all children – not only due to the many important substances contained in mother's milk, but also for the intimate contact. Sweet things or sugar obviously can't replace this love and care. They just reinforce the discontentment even more, since the emotional emptiness remains.

The need for love and bodily contact expresses itself in *Saccharum* children by behaviors such as thumb-sucking, nail-biting (including the toenails), and the demand to be carried or rocked. While one child might seek bodily contact, another might have difficulty accepting touch or caresses. Another way of getting attention is to be constantly asking questions or talking about something. When they want something, it must be IMMEDIATELY, since they're extremely impatient.

Poor concentration

When they don't get what they want, *Saccharum* children can become very furious, provocative, jealous, and aggressive. They demand attention by hitting, kicking, throwing things around, or behaving like a clown. They pull out all the stops to get what they want. They feel neglected and make quite sure that everyone else knows this.

A further problem is their concentration. They're very easily distracted, since they always want to look at and grab everything. Even the smallest things can distract their attention. They can only find peace when they learn to respect themselves, since deep inside they feel shy and unsure of themselves, and are yearning for the warmth and security of a good home. Longing is common in *Saccharum* children. They interpret criticism as a confirmation of their negative self-image. They're longing for some positive confirmation! Homeopathy can obviously not replace upbringing, but homeopathic remedies can help to heal old wounds. That's the goal.

Physical symptoms

Saccharum children have pale skin and a slight body-build, but there are also cases of the opposite, since they either eat too much or too little. At a later age too, *Saccharum* can help people with eating disorders if a lack of attention is the underlying cause.

Eczema is common in *Saccharum* children. They can also suffer from various inflammations, especially in the nose, throat, sinuses, and ears. When the children are somewhat older, they can even get diabetes mellitus or hypoglycemia (low blood sugar). Mouth ulcers (aphthae) and a tendency to get worms are particular indications for this remedy.

The Sepia Child

Contents of the ink sac of the common cuttlefish, Sepia officinalis (mollusc)

Animal remedy

"Dancing through life"

Origin

Sepia is a small sea creature similar to a squid that is found in coastal waters off Europe and Africa. In southern Europe, this cuttlefish is a speciality. *Sepia* is also known for its inner shell, which is used as an abrasive stone to trim the beaks of caged birds. The ink of sepia has been used since time immemorial to write and paint. The name sepia is also given to the dark brown shading similar to the ink, which we know from old photographs.

Hahnemann came across this remedy rather by chance. Although the Romans had used it medicinally, by his time it had fallen out of use as a medicine. One of his patients was an artist who suffered from all sorts of physical symptoms. Together they searched for the cause of these complaints. As Hahnemann watched the artist at work with sepia ink, it struck him that he repeatedly wet his brush with his tongue. Hahnemann suspected the culprit was something in the ink. By careful investigation of this substance, he discovered the great healing power of *Sepia*.

Sepia is one of the most well-known homeopathic remedies and is often used for menopausal complaints. It's less well known that it's also a suitable remedy for children.

Independent

Sepia children are generally independent from an early age, even though they might seem to be rather sensitive and delicate. When you first meet them, they're similar to *Phosphorus* children, since they're open and sensitive. But in contrast to *Phosphorus* children, they're good at keeping busy on their own and don't necessarily need other people.

They know what they want and are similar in many respects to *Nux vomica* children. They are strong-willed, full of energy, and temperamental. At first encounter, they act in an open and spontaneous way, yet as time goes on it becomes clear that they won't show their true feelings. Only in a safe environment do they open up completely and reveal their innermost secrets. But they can talk very enthusiastically about less intimate things!

Sense of rhythm

Even when they're very young, it's noticeable that they immediately start dancing when they hear music. They have an astonishing sense of rhythm. This is a clear difference from *Nux vomica* children, who don't show this unmistakable need for movement. If *Sepia* children are invited to a party, they may be reluctant to go, but as soon as the dancing starts, the mood changes abruptly. The desire to dance and the way it cheers them up is something we see in various homeopathic remedies, such as *Carcinosinum*. In general, *Sepia* children like to be physically active and this is when they are at their happiest. Apart from reading and playing music, these children should certainly play some kind of sport or do some kind of dancing!

Strong relationship with mother

Sepia is often prescribed in the clinic for girls. This can be due to the fact that it's harder to recognize in boys, and the physical symptoms are clearer in girls. *Sepia* girls frequently have a noticeably strong bond with their mother, which apparently contradicts their independence. If their mother is also a "*Sepia* mother," it can sometimes give the impression of Siamese twins — mother and daughter as an inseparable duo, who also look alike physically. Although we need to be careful when describing certain physical characteristics of a remedy picture, it's noticeable that *Sepia* children often have dark hair, especially when they get older.

Sensitive and snippy

They aren't weepy but when they're worried about something, it's best to leave them alone. They certainly don't want comfort, but prefer instead to retreat to their room. We can see certain characteristics of the cuttlefish in *Sepia* children. When they feel threatened, they either flee or go on the attack. When they're older, they can develop a pretty sharp tongue, and their fierce words are like the ink that the cuttlefish spurts out. They don't quickly forget injuries. Even when they've been quiet about something for a long time, they can suddenly and effortlessly "strike" someone at their most sensitive spot. They seem to possess a kind of sixth sense for this! Like *Phosphorus* children, *Sepia* children have a good understanding of people, but they tend not to share people's suffering.

Loneliness

They appear stubborn and independent, but in fact this is their way of protecting themselves against deeper hurts. When they don't feel recognized and loved, a feeling of loneliness develops. In contrast to *Phosphorus* children, they don't have the ability to directly express their feelings. They're reserved, the more so if their feelings were once hurt. *Sepia* helps them to heal the injury and become warm and open to other people.

Physical symptoms

Sepia children easily feel chilly and have a strong desire for warmth and sun. They're real sun worshippers! They have difficulty getting out of bed in the morning, but are all the more lively in the evening. Apart from headaches and abdominal pains, we also see neck, nose, and ear problems as well as skin complaints in *Sepia* children. The skin is often dry and can also be liable to fever blisters around the mouth. Many *Sepia* children have warts. A sallow complexion is characteristic for *Sepia*. When young girls already have a vaginal discharge, *Sepia* is one of the remedies to consider.
Physical exercise restores their energy balance.

Food and Drink

There's often a particularly strong desire for chocolate. They also like sweet things, spicy foods, and sour food. *Sepia* children mostly don't like fat and can't tolerate it well.

The Silicium Child

Silicon (Si)

Mineral remedy

"Slight but tough"

Origin

Until recently, we only prescribed *Silicea* (silicon dioxide). Now we also often prescribe pure silicon, known homeopathically as *Silicium*. Silicon is one of the most common elements on earth. Almost all rock contains at least some of this element. It can be said to form the earth's crust. The name *Silicium* comes from the Latin "silex" (pebble).

Silicon is very widely used. The durability of stone houses is due to their silicon-based compounds. It's added during the manufacture of steel structures to make it more flexible. Silicon is the most important element in semiconductor technology and is used, among other things, for the manufacture of computer microchips. The most important application is undoubtedly as a component of glass in the glass industry.

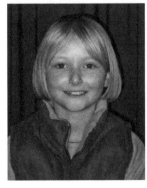

Sil.

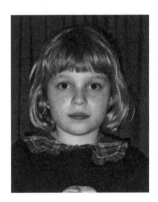

Sil.

In our bodies, silicon also plays an important role. It provides stable bones and firm connective tissue. A lack of silicon results in lifeless hair, brittle nails, and wounds that heal poorly.

Conscientious about detail

Silicium children have a keen sense of perception and a good intellect. They also have strong intuition and an eye for detail. Like *Phosphorus* children, they can easily sympathize with how someone feels, but they don't necessarily let this show, since they don't like putting themselves forward. They generally get on with people in a calm and straightforward way, but they can also be very stubborn when they have a different opinion about something. At school, they learn easily and are particularly good at mathematics. They can assimilate information quickly, know a lot, and retain everything they've learned, especially the details. They're very conscientious in this way. Moreover, they always give their best and work very precisely.

Fine and sensitive

Silicium children generally behave in a fine and aristocratic way. And their mostly delicate body build corresponds to this behavior. When they come from a stable family, they're well-balanced children. They can, therefore, be a support to other children, without taking on a leading role. They are sure of themselves because they've worked everything out down to the last detail. *Silicium* children are very conscientious.

They would like to leave a good impression, not so much of themselves as of what they do. The picture that other people have of them is important to them. They do the best they can, mindful of their reputation, and leave nothing to chance. This is another of the reasons for their precision.

Mild and non confrontational

Another characteristic of *Silicium* that we find in children is yielding. Although they stand up for their own opinion and can sometimes even be impertinent, they rarely get into arguments, preferring to yield rather than let it come to an argument. If they have a different opinion, they often prefer to keep it to themselves. This can make them seem quite reserved.

Sensitive to external influences

Silicium children are very sensitive. They sense what is going on in other people, and sometimes know things without being told. Many of them even have clairvoyant abilities. They're over-sensitive to influences from the environment, such as noise. Due to their delicacy of feeling, they can easily become disturbed, especially in terms of their self-confidence. This can be connected with the relationship they have with their father or the father figure in their life.

Shy

If they've become disturbed for any reason, they tend to withdraw more and become shy. Then they avoid all situations in which they have to prove themselves, such as tests, exams, and important meetings. They feel vulnerable and fragile. But other fears can come to the fore. *Silicium* children are typically afraid of sharp instruments such as pins, needles, and even ballpoint pens if someone is pointing one at them. Figuratively, this can be seen as a feeling of vulnerability. A single false word can destroy their carefully cultivated image in the same way that a small stone can destroy an entire window.

To avoid mistakes, with their inevitable emotional hurt, they work extremely conscientiously. The disadvantage is that they lose a sense of the whole due to their fixation on the details. Every mistake that other people find in what they do undermines their self-confidence. If these children are given *Silicium*, their self-confidence is strengthened and their general condition improves. This helps them to become reliable and dependable for others — as solid as a rock.

Physical symptoms

The bodies of *Silicium* children are not particularly well developed – they're slender and more susceptible to illness than other children. The intellect, on the other hand, is more strongly developed than in many other children. Even in small children we can see that their head is proportionally larger than their body. *Silicium* children often

211

suffer from colds that easily become ear infections or infections of the jaw or sinuses. It's typical for *Silicium* children that the glands sometimes become as hard as stone.

They easily get chilly and have many complaints due to cold.

When these children become ill, the *Silicium* metabolism in their body often starts malfunctioning. This can result in the hair and nails becoming brittle, wounds healing poorly, problems with the teeth, as well as disturbances of bone growth.

In puberty, they often suffer from acne, which can be cured with the homeopathic remedy *Silicium*. One of the complaints that we often hear of in *Silicium* children is sweaty feet. *Silicium* can also help here if the whole picture fits.

Food and Drink

The aversion to milk can be so great that *Silicium* children even reject breast milk, the best food there is. They usually can't tolerate milk and fat. *Silicium* children also don't like salt, meat, or warm food. They like eating eggs (though preferably with salt) and prefer cold food. *Silicium* children can also find sand tasty, which isn't so astounding because sand consists largely of silicon.

Silicium in the Clinic

Ruud's otorrhea

Ruud was six years old and had been suffering since birth from frequent bouts of otorrhea, which mostly affected the right ear and only occasionally the left. Apart from that, he suffered from abdominal complaints when he was tense. Ruud had very poor teeth that decayed when he was quite young.

At school, he was extremely popular – he always had many friends and was the "boss." He decided which games were to be played and who could play. He was an intelligent boy who behaved responsibly. He was very careful with his own things.

His mother said, however, that inside he was very uncertain of himself. He didn't let it show, but he was always afraid of making mistakes. With public events – such as a puppet theater – he tended to withdraw. He expressed anger only occasionally, and exactly as when afraid or in pain, he tended to withdraw.

Ruud easily got chilly and had few obvious food preferences. It was noticeable that he sweated heavily as he slept.

Due to the ear complaints and the combination of a domineering nature with uncertainty, I initially prescribed *Lycopodium*. After six weeks, there was no reaction at all. The fear of failure had if anything increased. So I gave him *Silicium*. Not only his ear complaints but also his mood then improved, and overall he felt much more at ease!

Due to a recurrence of his ear complaints, I later gave him another dose of *Silicium*. When I saw him six months later, he had had no further problems and felt better than ever before. According to his mother, he had become a different child with much more self-confidence and his mood was much better.

The Staphisagria Child

Stavesacre, Lice-Bane (Delphinium staphisagria)

Plant remedy (Ranunculaceae family)

"Magnanimous and vulnerable"

Origin

The members of the Ranunculaceae family, which include *Aconitum* and *Pulsatilla*, share a clear common picture. They feel abandoned and alone. They look for harmony with other people in order to overcome this feeling. They're very sensitive to rudeness. People should respect and be fond of each other, and avoid inflicting hurt. This delicacy is something we find even in very young children. One of their mottos in life is to accept the suffering of the world as it is, with all the associated toughness and lack of respect.

Dioscorides, the Roman doctor, used the seeds of this plant to induce vomiting and salivation. He also used it for toothache. In traditional medicine, *Delphinium staphisagria* was used as an ointment to kill lice. Hahnemann knew of this custom and pointed out that *Staphisagria* could be far more valuable as a homeopathic remedy.

Staphisagria is a biennial plant with violet flowers on stalks growing up to one meter high. The genus *"Delphinium"* comes from the Greek word "delphis," Latin "delphinus," which means "dolphin." The name refers to the shape of the flower, which is like a dolphin.

Sensitive

Staphisagria children are sensitive. They can sense how someone else is feeling, and they often have clairvoyant qualities. They're also extremely sensitive to how other people deal with them. In a pleasant and harmonious environment, they're cheerful and warmhearted with the sensitivity and playfulness of a dolphin.

But when they're hurt — and that happens very easily — quite a different side of their character comes to light. In their fury, they have fits of rage and throw things around, although not directly at other people, since they don't want to hurt anyone. They do this from a

214

feeling of powerlessness: "How can people do something like that to me?"

When they're very small, they can't express this in words, but you can see the outrage and horror in their faces. Simply comforting them doesn't do any good. They want their anger to be taken seriously. They want the other person to understand what's hurt them and to sympathize with them about it.

Lovable and vulnerable

The older they get, the more careful they become and the less they reveal of themselves. They have learnt the hard way that not everyone is as sensitive as they are, so now they try to protect themselves from the tough outside world. They do this by withdrawing when something is unpleasant for them. On the outside, they're normally lovable and obliging. That's their style, but it's also a way of avoiding getting hurt.

It's also true that they like to be seen as lovable. They need the warmth of others. And they also want other people to get on with each other in an affectionate way. Yet this doesn't mean that they'll put up with anything, since inside there's the same vulnerability and explosiveness!

Respect!

Staphisagria children have a high opinion of themselves. They want to be seen and respected, which can sometimes make them seem rather arrogant.

When they're at ease, they're naturally respected for their authority. In a school class or in a club, they're often elected to be the leader or representative. In this role, they can be very likable and behave respectfully and with feeling towards other people. Then they will certainly make sure that the children also treat each other respectfully. But there's a Dutch saying: "High trees catch much wind." In this exposed position, they're vulnerable to attack. Other power-hungry children will try to challenge them, and not always kindly.

Proud

When *Staphisagria* children get hurt, they either talk about it straight-away, becoming very vehement in the process – which is something they prefer to avoid – or they suppress the anger. Then it can take them a long time to get round to speaking about it. It's very important that parents take this into account and encourage their *Staphisagria* children to express their anger, since repressed feelings and hurt pride can really make them ill. Most complaints of *Staphisagria* children have to do with repressed emotions.

Their problem is that they would rather stand up for other people than for themselves. They have difficulty appreciating that children can be rough and unfair with each other, and they suffer accordingly. They would like to do something about it, but they often lack the strength or courage to actually intervene.

Children with this picture — whatever physical complaints they might have — need the homeopathic remedy *Staphisagria*. This remedy helps them settle down so that they find the courage to express themselves clearly and to face up to the necessary confrontation, without neglecting their sensitivity to other people.

Physical symptoms

Various complaints such as headaches, stomach pains, and diarrhea can arise if they don't express their anger. If the anger remains for a long time, the complaints can worsen, physically as well as psychologically.

Physical injuries after an operation, a bladder catheterization, or a cystoscopy (bladder scope) can be also cured by *Staphisagria*. It's known that many people get an infection after a bladder catheterization. *Staphisagria* would be the remedy of choice for this.

Eye complaints — styes and cysts - are also typical for this homeopathic remedy.

Food and Drink

Staphisagria children love spicy food and cold milk. Older children can have a strong desire to smoke, which should obviously be discouraged. Otherwise they immediately get problems.

The Stramonium Child

Thorn apple, Jimson weed (Datura stramonium)

Plant remedy (Solanaceae family)

"Alone in the dark woods"

Origin

The thorn apple is a plant that's now so common in Europe that it probably seems to be indigenous. Yet history shows that the thorn apple was introduced from America by the Spanish doctor, Francisco Hernandez, more than 400 years ago. The alkaloids that it contains – hyoscyamine, atropine, and scopolamine — are still used nowadays in medicine. The whole plant was very popular in former times due to its hallucinogenic qualities, but was rarely used in this form because it's extremely poisonous. It was also used for emotional agitation, asthma, and cramps. As a homeopathic remedy, it can also relieve these kinds of illnesses and often heal them too. The Solanaceae (nightshade) family also includes the homeopathic remedies *Belladonna* and *Hyoscyamus*.

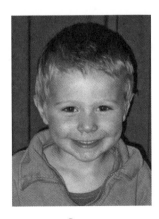

Stram.

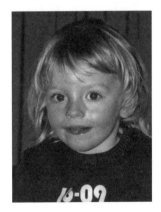

Stram.

Fear of the dark

Stramonium children or children who temporarily enter the Stramonium state are certainly afraid of the dark. They are, therefore, afraid of tunnels, which is a strong indication for this remedy. Obviously, there are several types of children who are afraid of the dark, but it's unmistakable in Stramonium. They can react with panic if there's not at least one small light on! They have dreadful visions of everything that could happen to them. It's not uncommon for dangerous animals to appear in their fantasies — for example, big black dogs attacking them — as well as monsters and people who want to harm them. When there's a nightlight on and they know that their parents are nearby, they feel safe.

When Stramonium children are ill, they can suddenly wake up at night in complete panic. Then they want to go into their parents' bed or to be carried by them.

The fear is very similar to the feeling of suddenly being alone in the jungle or in the darkness. The sounds of wild animals are all around and death is lurking everywhere. A typical fear found above all in Stramonium children is fear of water.

Flight or fight

Their reaction to fear is flight or fight. Even in their day-to-day dealings, their behavior is usually extreme. When they're cheerful, they can be really hearty, but the behavior they show when afraid is very distinctive. If parents or older people are nearby, Stramonium children will try and cling to them. If no one is nearby, they can even go on the attack, like a cornered animal. In their fear, they can sometimes even fail to recognize their own parents, especially on waking from a nightmare. It's possible, therefore, that a parent gets scratched or hit.

In their aggression, they break things, spit, or throw objects. Although this is driven by fear, it can sometimes appear to outsiders like a groundless tantrum. At school, at home, or in the neighborhood, Stramonium children can cause a lot of damage when they feel threatened.

Restless children

In a similar way to Belladonna children, Stramonium children can be very restless and can, therefore, find themselves being quickly pigeonholed as suffering from Attention-Deficit Hyperactivity Disorder (ADHD). For example, they run to and fro, climb over everything, turn everything upside down, make a racket, then play the clown again, tell endless stories, or sing songs. As far as singing is concerned, they're similar to *Hyoscyamus* children, even if these are mostly much more jealous. Incidentally, there are several possible remedies for ADHD — see the chapter "Restless Children in the Clinic."

They have a noticeably high pain threshold. Exactly like *Opium* children, they seem to be scarcely sensitive to pain in this wild state. Their bodies can also move grotesquely, in a dance-like or a strained and cramped way.

As already mentioned, the fear is caused mostly by the darkness, but when they're overexcited, *Stramonium* children can also be annoyed by bright light, mirrors, and reflective objects.

Physical symptoms

Hahnemann stated that the most impressive symptoms are to be found on the psychological level. On the physical level, cramps are the most obvious symptom. These can be twitches in the face as well as cramp-like movements of the arms and legs, or even the whole body, as in epilepsy. Asthma attacks that begin at night, causing the child to panic in the dark, are very specific for *Stramonium*. Asthma can also be seen as a kind of cramp.

When the cramps occur in the abdomen, they're mostly very severe — in this case, we certainly don't see the high pain threshold mentioned earlier.

The tendency to cramps also expresses itself in the voice: many *Stramonium* children stutter, especially when they're excited. Physical symptoms in *Stramonium* children can worsen due to fear, fever, and too much sun.

Food and Drink

Although they can be very thirsty, it's striking that they sometimes have a horror of drinking — as if they were afraid of it.

They can also find that everything tastes bitter.

Stramonium in the Clinic

Homeopathy can help to heal emotional traumas

Bert was an athletic youth of 17 who had been suffering from depression for several years. Now and then, it got so bad that he would rather be dead! He had fantasies of how he could end his life. What's more, he was extremely irritable — even the sound of someone biting an apple could drive him crazy.

The deep depression had begun when he injured himself after a very successful sporting year — he was one of the best at his sport in the Netherlands. For years, sport had been his emotional outlet, and he had been marvelously successful. The passion for sport had originated one year earlier. At this time, he had gone into a high-school class in which he became the whipping boy. In contrast to his fellow pupils, he was serious and liked learning. He was abused and harassed.

To get rid of the suppressed aggression, he threw himself into sport, with great success! After a few years, the harassment ceased but the scars remained. He couldn't tolerate any contact, and he felt threatened by everything. He slept poorly and was regularly woken up abruptly by dreadful dreams. Bert also had some physical complaints. He frequently suffered from headaches and warmth made him dizzy.

Due to the feeling of being threatened and the inner aggressiveness, I decided to prescribe him a dose of *Stramonium*. Within a few weeks, an improvement set in, and after two months he said that he felt well. The irritability had disappeared, and when he thought of the past, it didn't disturb him so much. The remedy had helped him to work through the disturbing incidents. He still occasionally suffered from headaches, especially due to temperature changes, but the dizziness had disappeared.

After another dose of *Stramonium*, his condition improved further. The last time I saw him — four months after the first consultation — he felt well in every way and no longer had headaches.

The Sulfur Child

Sulfur (S)

Mineral remedy

"It's marvelous to be loved!"

Origin

In the past, *Sulfur* was one of the most frequently prescribed homeopathic remedies. Not only because we knew what type it suited, but also because of its wide spectrum of action. *Sulfur* is worth considering for many complaints. In the last ten years, however, the picture of *Sulfur* has become much clearer. It remains one of our most important remedies, but it works best when the whole picture fits the child as well as possible.

Sulfur is mostly found in compounds with other elements. In many places, for example near Naples, there have been sulfur springs since time immemorial, where we find this element in an exceptionally pure form. Since sulfur is flammable at low temperatures, it was used in the past to light fires. An example of this is "The Little Match Girl" (the title of a fairy tale by Hans Christian Andersen) — the matches in the story were made of sulfur.

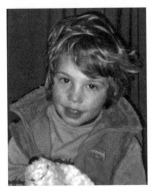

Sulf.

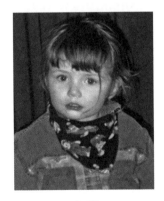

Sulf.

221

Nowadays we use phosphorus to make matches, since sulfur catches fire too easily. It's no coincidence that phosphorus and sulfur are next to each other in the periodic table. These two chemical elements have many similarities such as fieriness and high flammability, but there are also differences.

In our bodies, sulfur is an important trace element, contained in proteins and enzymes among other things.

Need for intimate contact

Sulfur fits the period of children's lives when they're seeking a relationship and trying to discover themselves. While *Phosphorus* children mostly have many friends in order to feel connected, *Sulfur* children tend to be looking for a single person with whom they can share their innermost feelings. They're particularly concerned with the feeling of being loved and experiencing the love that the other person feels for them. As long as they can't find this in another person, they don't mind being alone. In contrast to *Phosphorus* children, they don't necessarily need other people.

Sulfur children really flourish in an atmosphere of love and harmony, and then they can share their charm and their love with others. That's exactly what they're after: relationships in which they can give and receive love in equal parts.

Sense of beauty

When relationships are forming, external appearance plays a key role. This is why *Sulfur* children pay special attention to it. They love fine clothes and can be very critical in this respect. They know exactly which pair of trousers or which dress is in fashion and refuse to wear anything else. Young *Sulfur* girls show off in their best clothes; *Sulfur* boys make sure that their appearance fits their image. The aim is always to be loved. That's their deepest wish.

But other impressions are also important when a relationship is developing. Smell, for example, plays a major role here. Just think of perfume! Even young *Sulfur* children have a strong preference for certain smells. If they smell something unpleasant, they can sometimes feel sick.

Researcher and collector

Exactly like *Phosphorus* children, *Sulfur* children have a strong thirst for knowledge. When they're small, they want to grab hold of everything — "looking with the hands." When they're somewhat older, they want to know everything and can become engrossed in a particular object of study.

If they possess a stamp collection, it has to be complete, and they'll collect every stamp they can find. They can, however, suddenly lose interest. When something doesn't interest them, they neglect it completely. This is exactly the same as their relationship to people: it's all about one thing or one person. Their interest can be on the intellectual level — that's their main strength — but also on the practical level. In this case, they love taking things apart and putting them back together again. They can completely lose themselves doing this.

Jealousy and fantasy

The love of other people, their parents, their siblings, and their friends, supports their self-love. Yet when they miss a person's love and have the feeling that someone else is receiving more of that person's love than they are, this feels to them like a rebuff. They quickly feel unloved, which can lead to jealousy. They then try – for example, by showy clothes or bad behavior — to attract the attention and love that they're missing.

In their frustration, they can become really nasty. The element Sulfur is very easily flammable and *Sulfur* children too can become furious at the slightest opportunity. Or they sometimes just withdraw. They become quiet, want to be alone, and then lose themselves in their private fantasies. They are prone to flights of fantasy, but the danger is that they dream up images and expectations that have no connection with reality, which invariably leads to disappointment.

Indifference

If *Sulfur* children find that love doesn't "flow" in a natural way, they become indifferent. Indifference is a defense mechanism. It conceals sadness and loneliness. They try to use their thoughts to suppress their emotions, so that they no longer have to feel, and this often works only too well. Yet it means they lose their "joie de vivre." In this phase, they can become critical and possibly also cynical. No one loves them and they don't even care. It can go so far that they neglect their appearance and no longer want to wash themselves.

We also find this symptom in *Ammonium carbonicum* children, especially when they're angry or hurt. They can then withdraw completely and want to have nothing to do with anyone.

Physical symptoms

The main reason why *Sulfur* children visit a homeopathic doctor is for skin complaints. *Sulfur* fits all kinds of skin disease, especially where there is itching. The skin is dry and itchy, worsening with warmth (especially the warmth of the bed) and water.

Burning is a symptom running right through the *Sulfur* picture. After the scratching, the skin begins to burn. Burning pains can also occur anywhere else on the body. The body has "fire inside," which is why *Sulfur* children easily get too warm. For this reason they stick their feet out from under the bedclothes. Almost all complaints get worse with warmth.

We don't often notice the typical *Sulfur* smell (like rotten eggs) in children, but *Sulfur* children do have a strong body odor, especially when they're feeling unwell.

Their digestion is rapid. Even when they've had a good breakfast, they need to eat something at 11:00 and again at 16:00 (4 p.m.), despite having eaten at midday. If they don't regularly eat, they can start to feel really bad. The gut is generally a weak spot for *Sulfur* children.

Food and Drink

Sulfur children love spicy food, with herbs if possible, but certainly with a distinctive taste. They also love sweet things, olives and fat, although they can't tolerate this very well. They either like or dislike milk and meat.

Sulfur in the Clinic

Wim's colds

Wim was not quite two years old when he came to see me with his parents. From birth on, he had had colds with a lot of mucus. Above all, his parents were shocked when the audiological clinic diagnosed a serious hearing impairment. Several months before the consultation, he had had his adenoids removed, but this had hardly brought any improvement. Shortly afterwards, he had another inflammation of the middle ear on both sides, and then a few weeks before coming to see me he had had two further closely spaced episodes of inflammation of the left ear.

On the father's side of the family, colds were common. His father had also frequently had bronchitis in the past.

Wim's appetite was good except when he was ill. Then he ate virtually nothing. He was always thirsty. His desire for sweet things was noticeable as well as his aversion to eggs. At night he was like a "whirlwind," constantly tossing and turning in bed. He didn't really need a cover on his bed. His stool was always slightly thin.

As far as his character was concerned, he had a strong will and a need for particular patterns. He was always putting things straight if they were hanging or standing at an angle. He had an eye for that. He had a strong desire to be active, and he investigated anything new. Shyness or fear couldn't stop him doing this. If something interested him, he "looked at it with his hands." He went up to everything — including other children — and could stand up for himself well. If other children tried to take something off him, he raged and screamed and would even hit out. He was very determined when dealing with grown-ups. He looked at people briefly and then decided whether he liked them or not. Despite his tendency to put things in their place, he could cause a fair amount of chaos.

Due to his physical complaints and his character, I decided to prescribe him *Sulfur*. The reaction was spectacular. After a week, he had one last brief cold and then no more. His breathing, which had always been heavy, became normal again. He went to sleep far more easily and calmly, and his hearing improved markedly.

225

In the space of a few weeks, he began to talk again. When I examined his ears, I found that the Eustachian tube was clear on both sides, which significantly reduced the probability of another infection.

Hans' ear infections

Hans had been sick a lot as a baby, and the ear infections had started from the eighth month. Apart from that, he almost always had a cold, which always turned into a middle-ear infection. Up to that point, he had had one course of antibiotics from the family doctor, but his parents wanted Hans to be treated homeopathically to strengthen his resistance to illness.

When I saw Hans for the first time, he had just had his first birthday. He was a jolly fellow, cheeky, mischievous, and quick-tempered. He was afraid of nothing and was very active. His mood could change abruptly. One moment he was laughing, the next he was crying over some triviality, yet he did accept consolation well.

Due to his warm-blooded nature, his physical complaints, and his character, I gave him *Pulsatilla*. As a result, his complaints improved, although he remained susceptible and his behavior became if anything more boisterous.

When he was four years old, his mother brought him again. In the meantime, he had started elementary school. *Pulsatilla* had improved his immune system but he was still susceptible and was currently going through another phase of chronic coughing. His mother explained how he was untidy and would frequently hit out when angry. Due to his character together with his known dislike of eggs and milk, I decided to prescribe him *Sulfur*. Now a positive change came over him at all levels. His behavior became calmer, it was easier to talk to him, and he felt physically better.

Not until a year later was another dose of *Sulfur* necessary, and the improvement held right through the following year, both on the psychological and physical level.

The Thuja occidentalis Child

Tree of life

Plant remedy (Cupressaceae family)

"Searching for your roots"

Origin

This remedy is prepared from a tincture of the fresh green twigs of the eastern tree of life. A long time ago, it was given the name "tree of life" (in Latin, "arbor vitae"), which says a lot about its ability to restore our life energy. Originally, the tree of life only grew in the northern United States and Canada. In the middle of the 18th century, it was imported to France. Due to its naturally perfect conical shape, it's used for high hedges. It has a characteristically thick leaf covering, through which the stem is not visible. The tree can live for over a thousand years, and its wood is used for coffins, among other things.

Before Hahnemann, there was little information about the healing effects of this tree. The famous 18th century Dutch doctor, Baerhaave, reported on the effectiveness of the sap in illnesses where edema occurs. In the United States, *Thuja* is used as an herbal remedy for pain in the limbs. The symptoms mentioned also fit the homeopathic remedy picture.

Vaccination problems

In the past, *Thuja* was the homeopathic remedy of choice for complaints following vaccination. It was only common to vaccinate against smallpox in the past, and since *Thuja* is one of the main remedies for skin abscesses, it's not surprising that *Thuja* can in many cases heal the effects of vaccinations.

A chance discovery

One of Hahmenann's patients prompted him to come up with the idea of making a homeopathic remedy from this tree. The patient was a priest who had all sorts of complaints that Hahnemann

227

couldn't classify. Like a detective, Hahnemann followed everything the priest did to try and find the cause of his mysterious symptoms. Eventually he found the culprit. As he wandered around reading his prayer book, the unhappy priest always passed by a *Thuja* tree and absentmindedly plucked a twig. He put this in his mouth and started chewing it – and this was the source of his problems!

Dreamy and sensitive

Thuja children can be very dreamy, as if they haven't quite made it down to earth. They're by nature very sensitive to particular moods. The impression people make, the prevailing mood in a house, or music – absolutely anything can move them deeply. This sensitivity means they're often artistically gifted, in music as well as in writing and poetry.

The toughness of daily life quickly overwhelms them and they have the feeling that they need to protect themselves. Their reaction can be to completely close themselves off, which is a pattern reminiscent of autism. In this respect, they're similar to *Helium* children. *Thuja* helps these children to discover their own roots and thereby also their own feelings.

Vulnerable

It's important for *Thuja* children to be accepted as they are. By nature, they're very sensitive and so are easily hurt. The inner vulnerability of *Thuja* children is best illustrated by the feeling of "being made of glass." Obviously, this feeling is rarely articulated as such. The feeling "being made of glass" expresses how fragile and vulnerable someone is. In addition, glass is transparent – *Thuja* children feel as if other people can see straight through them. When they become unsettled, they can find it unbearable to be touched or looked at.

Difficulties with change

The fear of the unknown and of strangers means that any change is very difficult for them and can upset their equilibrium.

On the outside, *Thuja* children appear very strong, which does in fact correspond to their inner steadfastness and stamina. They are sometimes, however, very discontented with themselves and can doubt their self-worth. One possible cause of this is that they were unwanted children. A further cause can be that unreasonable demands are made of them, which they then try to fulfill — for example, the daughter of a father who would rather have had a son, or the child used by a couple to try and get over the death of their other child. Moreover, earlier traumas that prevented the development of the child's own identity can cause the child to enter a *Thuja* state.

Shutting off and hardening

The only way these children have of defending themselves is to shut off, a reaction that reminds us of *Natrium muriaticum* children. Outwardly they adapt as well as possible since they know exactly what's expected of them. Other people, therefore, have the impression that they aren't really being themselves and that they're not behaving as they really are — as if they were carrying a secret around inside.
Driven by their inner urge to survive, which is very strong, they tend to harden themselves. Their feelings change into a kind of fanaticism. They can become dogmatic and, for example, sport can become their main goal in life. They throw themselves with such diligence into their work that they easily forget the original reason for what they're doing. Minor details become more important than the whole. We also see this issue in *Silicium* children.
The hardening is connected with the need for control. By sticking to what's familiar, they know where they are. *Calcarea carbonica* children also show this tendency. Changes can easily unsettle them, not just external changes such as a move or a new school, but also inner changes such as during puberty. The fear of the unknown can be so great that they begin to tremble in the presence of strangers.

Own identity

Since they've often learned as very young children to deny their own feelings and to bow to the expectations of others, it's difficult for *Thuja* children to be themselves and to develop their own identity. Who am I really? *Thuja* helps these children to be themselves again and to find out what they want – to work out who they really are.

Physical symptoms

Most physical complaints affect the left side of the body, the feeling side. It is, after all, feelings that *Thuja* children all too easily suppress. They can even have the feeling that their body and soul are separated. In general, *Thuja* children react poorly to cold damp weather and their complaints worsen at 03:00 and 15:00
(3 a.m. and 3 p.m.).

The way the body reacts is very characteristic for *Thuja*: wart-like outgrowths, flaky skin and fever rash round the mouth, malformations of the nails, and various hardenings frequently occur. The skin can react with increased sweating, especially under the armpits, in the pubic area, and on the upper lip.

Along with *Natrium sulfuricum*, *Thuja* is the main remedy for asthma that worsens in cold damp weather. Pounding headaches, as if nails were being hammered in, especially on the left side of the forehead, are typical for *Thuja*. Moreover, we also see joint problems and stiffness in *Thuja* children. The pains are worsened by stretching! The kidneys, the bladder, and the genitals are extremely sensitive.

Food and Drink

Thuja children don't like unusual food. As the Dutch saying goes, "What the farmer doesn't know, he doesn't eat." They can have a strong desire for chocolate. There's frequently a dislike of onions, fresh meat, and peppers. They often can't tolerate onions, tea, fat, and seasoned food.

The Tuberculinum Child

Nosode

"Burning the candle at both ends"

Origin

Until antibiotics were discovered, tuberculosis was an illness that also occurred frequently in the West. At that time, homeopathy was one of the few branches of medicine that was successful in treating this illness (together with rest and a healthy environment). Since people who had survived tuberculosis often continued to suffer from various other complaints for long periods, the doctors had the idea of preparing a homeopathic remedy from a culture of tuberculosis bacilli (*Mycobacterium tuberculosis*). Robert Koch had discovered this bacterium in 1882. After potentization (diluting and shaking), the homeopathic remedy no longer contains even a single molecule of the original substance — in other words, no bacteria remain. Homeopaths have gained much experience in the last 100 years using *"Tuberculinum Koch."* So now we know which complaints fit this remedy and also what type of person or child reacts best to it.

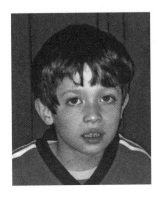

Tub.

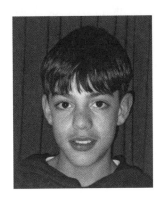

Tub.

231

Besides *Tuberculinum Koch*, there are many other strains of bacteria that are used as homeopathic remedies. To prepare *Tuberculinum Koch*, human or bovine strains are used. *Tuberculinum bovinum* Kent is made from the tubercular glands of slaughtered cattle, and *Tuberculinum aviaire* from a pathogenic culture of avian tuberculosis. The different forms all have similar modes of action

Important child remedy

There was a time when almost every child who was susceptible to colds or who had lung complaints was also prescribed *Tuberculinum*, so successful was this remedy. In the meantime, there are considerably more remedies that fit these symptoms, but *Tuberculinum* is still frequently prescribed for children. If we find inexplicable symptoms, and then we find out that tuberculosis occurs in the family history, we immediately think of this remedy.

But also for more well-known illnesses like allergies, chronic colds, and lung disease, *Tuberculinum* (for a limited period) can be necessary to strengthen the immune system. *Tuberculinum* fits the overall picture for some children. They don't just need this remedy for their physical well-being, but also for their emotional well-being. These are the true "*Tuberculinum* children."

Life's too short

When we watch how *Tuberculinum* children live, it seems as if they have too little time. Anything can catch their attention and they would really like to do several things at the same time. As long as they feel more or less happy, they make an open and spontaneous impression. They then resemble *Phosphorus* children and can be just as radiant. They find everything interesting and are open to everything. Due to their charming manner, they know how to easily win over other people. They love new things, new contacts, and new challenges. Nothing is too much for them. In this respect, they're completely different from *Calcarea carbonica* children, even if there are many similarities on the physical level.

Restless journey of discovery

The need for change and discovery can lead to discontent and restlessness. *Tuberculinum* is one of the homeopathic remedies that fit

Attention-Deficit Hyperactivity Disorder (ADHD). They can't sit still at all! Whether they want to or not, they register all kinds of external stimuli, which they then have to cope with. If *Tuberculinum* children encounter resistance, they tend to go on the attack, in contrast to *Carcinosinum* children, who would rather fit in. Their anger can turn into fits of rage: they throw things around, hit, scream, swear, and kick. They'll use any method to express their dissatisfaction. "No" is the only answer they give, even to a well-meaning question.

If this behavior doesn't lead to success, then they want to leave and go somewhere else. When they're angry, they can run very fast. Other children may be too fearful to leave their familiar surroundings, but not *Tuberculinum* children! As soon as they can walk, they make use of this mobility. Everything new is exciting, and traveling means everything to them.

Few fears

Tuberculinum children are difficult to impress. They mostly have considerable self-confidence. When everyone else has already given up hope, they can still see a glimmer of light. They aren't afraid of being punished and can even react to punishment with complete indifference. They know what they want (or what they don't want) and go right to the edge for it. If their discontent and restlessness grow, it can quickly lead to changeable moods and impulsivity.

What was initially a defiant reaction can turn into outright maliciousness. Then they can break things or hurt other children. They give the impression that they can't help themselves, that they're being driven by some inner force.

One of the few fears that we see in *Tuberculinum* is the fear of animals, especially dogs (sometimes also cats). It's possible that they see their own inner state reflected in the animals and it's this that they're really afraid of. At night, they're often very fearful, even if they can't say what it is they're afraid of.

Everything in a state of flux

The development of *Tuberculinum* children is rapid. Here too, it's as if they want to make full use of the time and not miss out on anything. Experimenting with various things such as drugs and sexuality is more common in *Tuberculinum* children than others. They're often sexually precocious, and here too they want to discover everything. Obviously, the overall picture must fit for us to prescribe *Tuberculinum*, as there are several remedies that fit precocious children. *Tuberculinum* children keep getting the feeling that life might be too short and that they have to experience everything NOW!

Physical symptoms

Although we should be cautious about physical characteristics, there are nevertheless some features that appear to be specific to *Tuberculinum*. The downy hair on the back of newborn babies, which normally disappears in a few days or at the most a few weeks, remains with *Tuberculinum* children noticeably longer, sometimes even a few years. From the observation of thousands of patients, it turns out that the eyelashes are longer than average. Noticeably red lips are an additional indication.

Night sweats and grinding of the teeth are symptoms that fit *Tuberculinum* (and *Belladonna*). If there's also an increased susceptibility to colds and lung complaints, or if there's even been pneumonia in the past, the choice of remedy is clear. *Tuberculosis* in an ancestor is an additional reason to prescribe this remedy. With colds, the adenoids enlarge and the lymph nodes in the neck swell up.

Tuberculinum children are sensitive to temperature changes. The results can include colds, airway infections, or also rheumatic complaints. In general, they like warm and dry weather, and it's important that they always get enough fresh air.

Tuberculinum children can react very negatively to things affecting the immune system, which is why it's advisable to be careful about immunizations.

Tuberculinum children often have skin complaints. It's noticeable that the itch gets stronger when the clothes have been removed and on contact with cold water, but improves with warmth. Allergies also fit the *Tuberculinum* picture.

During sleep, *Tuberculinum* children frequently move their head to and fro, and sometimes even ram the edge of the bed or the wall – just like the head-banging in their temper tantrums! At the sea and in the mountains, *Tuberculinum* children mostly feel better, and some complaints can even disappear there, as was often the case in the past for patients with tuberculosis!

Tuberculinum bovinum fits stomach and gut complaints whereas allergies to feathers are a strong indication for *Tuberculinum aviaire*.

Food and Drink

Tuberculinum children often have a great need for (cold) milk and ice cream. They also like fatty and seasoned food, as well as bananas, sweet things, and warm drinks.

There can be either a desire for or an aversion to meat and sour foods.

Tuberculinum in the Clinic

Gert's eczema

Gert was two years old and was suffering from eczema on his upper thighs and his thumb. The thumb caused him the most problems. Cracks would form regularly and they bled. He also had little appetite, which concerned his mother most of all. At regular intervals, he had a runny nose. Following a middle-ear infection, his sense of hearing was diminished.

His night sweats were noticeable. There were also many cases of eczema in the family.

Gert was a happy, open, and sharp-witted little fellow who could defend himself well. When he was angry, he yelled and stamped his feet, but this passed quickly. His enormous fear of animals was striking.

Due to the combination of night sweats, fear of animals, eczema, and colds, I prescribed him *Tuberculinum*. His reaction was quick and positive. The skin improved, and the remedy was repeated when the eczema reappeared a few weeks later. From this point on, he remained well. It was agreed with the parents to only give Gert a further dose of *Tuberculinum* if his complaints became acute.

Restless Children in the Clinic

There have always been restless children — children who can't sit still and are distracted by everything. This used to be known as Minimal Cerebral Dysfunction (MCD), whereas nowadays it's called Attention-Deficit Hyperactivity Disorder (ADHD) — at least, when the symptoms match all the criteria.

For a homeopathic doctor, restlessness in a child is always a symptom and never simply a diagnosis. By nature, there are many different temperaments. There are children who are very quiet or even phlegmatic, and there are children who like to be active and who find it difficult to sit still for long periods. There are children who are intellectually oriented and others who like to be physically active. Yet true ADHD is more than this. The restlessness of ADHD children is something that they themselves can't deal with. They need help.

Conventional medicine has come up with drugs (Ritalin, Adderall, Concerta and others), which are helpful in many cases. The children become calmer and can concentrate better, but is that the solution? These drugs obviously influence the central nervous system (CNS) — with what long-term effects? Homeopathy is a useful support in many cases and a real alternative for a lot of children.

A homeopathic doctor will try to get to the bottom of what's causing the symptoms. The search is very individual, but sometimes certain patterns are recognizable. The following are some examples of this.

Familial

Disposition and inheritance always play a role. A parent often says: "But that's how I was as a child!" Whereas someone's disposition luckily can't be changed, it is indeed possible to alter an imbalance that can be traced back to a particular disorder in the family. Investigations indicate that inheritance plays a role in three-quarters of the children with ADHD.

Tuberculosis is one possible cause of disorders that homeopaths know about. People often no longer realize that one of their ancestors had tuberculosis. On the one hand, it can be a long time ago; on the other hand, this illness was not discussed in the past. Home-

237

opathic doctors recognize the symptoms that belong to this disorder. The children have the feeling that their lives are too short and that they must experience everything before they die. Their behavior is accordingly very intense and restless. They always want to be doing or seeing something different or something new. They're open, spontaneous children, interested in everything, but they don't have the patience to occupy themselves with something for any length of time. *Tuberculinum*, the homeopathic remedy made from a culture of tuberculosis bacilli (yet there is not a single molecule of the original substance in the remedy), is a very important remedy in the treatment of ADHD. Other remedies that fit this issue are *Medorrhinum* and *Luesinum*.

Allergies

According to the nutritionists, around 10 % of children with ADHD are really suffering from a food allergy. There are various subtle methods that can be used to establish if there is an over-sensitivity to particular foods. Well-known foods that can cause restlessness are sugar, colorings, and flavorings. Children in general, not just those with ADHD, become more restless the more sugar they eat. It's therefore advisable to restrict the sugar intake of children as much as possible.

Environmental factors

When things happen in children's lives to unsettle them, an ADHD picture can arise. Examples are mistreatment, neglect, and abuse. Along with psychological assistance, homeopathy can help to stabilize children so that they can come to terms with these kinds of trauma.

Thanks to the work of the Dutch homeopathic doctor Jan Scholten, we've discovered a valuable remedy for many children who have been traumatized after the separation of their parents: *Magnesium muriaticum*. *Magnesium* is related to fear of losing someone and to suppressed anger. People who need a *Magnesium* compound repress their anger because they're afraid of losing the other person. *Muriaticum* (chloride) is related to the mother. The mother represents care and attention and is the most important person for the (small) child. Children who have just experienced their parents' separation often blame themselves, as if to say to themselves: "If you're bad, your mother or father will go away." Roughly speaking, there are two types of reaction: children who become quiet and try to avoid any discord; or the exact opposite, children who try to attract as much as attention as possible, rather like a lightning conductor for the parents' conflict. The latter group can be very unsettled. They do everything possible to draw attention to themselves, positively as well as negatively. After a dose of *Magnesium muriaticum*, we often see that these children are able to express their emotions so that they can let go of their anger and fear.

Learning problems

The expectations made of children these days are considerable, including intellectual performance at an ever earlier age. For children who are eager to learn and who are self-confident, this is not so much of a problem as for children who are somewhat slower at school or who are still too playful. The pressure felt by these children can cause them to doubt themselves. They do their best, but always have the feeling that they can't achieve what's expected. Sometimes this feeling can arise from something minor such as a chance remark by the teacher or a fellow pupil. The fear of being thought stupid is sadly common in adults too, usually due to an experience long ago at school.

Fortunately, there are also homeopathic remedies for these children, such as *Calcarea phosphorica* or *Barium phosphoricum*.

Children who need *Calcarea phosphorica* can be very similar to typical ADHD children. They have a hard time sitting still, find it difficult to concentrate, and are easily distracted.

In principle, there are hundreds of remedies that might suit a child with ADHD, remedies that can often be used with good success. In my experience the most common remedies include *Tuberculinum, Lithium phosphoricum, Belladonna, Sulphur, Agaricus, Tarentula, Medorrhinum, Cina, Chamomilla* and *Saccharum*.

Other factors

Medicines that the mother receives during pregnancy can reach the growing child and trigger a variety of symptoms. If a homeopathic remedy is made from the medicine, this can work wonders. Immunization can also cause behavioral changes in children. There are many well-known examples of this. In other words: work together with your homeopath to look for possible causes. There is often a suitable homeopathic remedy. Such cases are obviously not suitable for self-medication.

Ear and Eye Complaints in Children

Small children have ear complaints more often than older children and adults. That's because their Eustachian tubes (the connection between the middle ear and the pharynx) tend to lie horizontally. This means blockages are more likely, leading to infection. At this age, the adenoids and tonsils are often enlarged. Together with colds, this can lead to ear problems.

Ear infections

Most children have an ear infection at some time. This is often preceded by a cold, but the infection often begins suddenly and without previous symptoms. The infection can be accompanied by intense pain, which can easily be seen in the children's reactions. The way they react to the pain crucially informs the homeopath's decision for a particular remedy. Along with a nose spray to loosen the mucus, such a remedy can work wonders. The two most important remedies are *Chamomilla* and *Pulsatilla*. *Belladonna* can also be necessary, especially when the fever starts suddenly, as well as when there are febrile seizures.

Chamomilla picture

Children who need *Chamomilla* (chamomile) tolerate pain very poorly. When they're troubled by pains in the ears or teeth — for which the remedy is very often prescribed — they have raging fits. They scream and make an incredible noise, as if someone was mistreating them. Whatever the parents try, it's very hard to calm them down. They only calm down when they're carried and at the same time rocked. But woe betide the parents who stop doing this!
Chamomilla is one of the remedies that convince people of the efficacy of homeopathy, since it can very rapidly put an end to a child's pain.

Pulsatilla picture

Another remedy that's good for children with ear infections is *Pulsatilla* (small pasque flower). This type of child reacts quite differently to pain than *Chamomilla* children. They are and always will be mostly sweet and gentle. They try to attract more attention than normal and try to achieve this by softly crying so they'll be able to slip onto the lap of their mother or father. They have an enormous need for consolation! Any kind of consolation can help them and seems to soothe the pain. As soon as they've been left alone again, they feel like the most pathetic people in the world and start crying from self-pity. In short, after a dose of *Pulsatilla* they once again become happy and fun-loving.

Chronic ear infections and tubal catarrh

Children who often suffer from middle-ear infections or who have chronic tubal catarrh can develop so-called glue ear. If the Eustachian tubes continue to be blocked so that the middle ear cannot drain, the fluid in the middle ear thickens. Homeopathically, several remedies can provide relief, but sometimes it's advisable to have the doctor insert a grommet into the eardrum.

Eye complaints in newborn babies

All newborn babies used to be treated with silver nitrate eyedrops to prevent particular eye diseases. Nowadays, this procedure is no longer routinely performed, since the drops themselves can lead to irritation of the eyes. Many babies suffer in the first few weeks from "festering" eyes. Most forms are easy to treat but sometimes a homeopathic remedy is also necessary.

Inflammation of the eye

The whites of the eyes and the inside of the eyelids are covered with a mucous membrane, the conjunctiva. In most cases, inflammation of the eye is actually inflammation of the conjunctiva and is known as conjunctivitis. Conjunctivitis is not at all dangerous to the eye. A mild cold can cause the eye to discharge some light or colored mucus. If necessary, the eye can be cleansed with a cotton bud and some water (boiled and allowed to cool).

If the mucus is greenish or yellowish, it's better to consult a doctor. If the inflammation is painless and accompanied by a cold, it can be easily treated. If the inflammation is stubborn or recurs, the homeopathic doctor can look for a suitable remedy that fits the cold as well as the child's type. Frequently prescribed remedies in such cases include *Pulsatilla*, *Graphites*, and *Medorrhinum*.

Skin Complaints in the Clinic

For a homeopathic doctor, skin complaints are the body's signal that something isn't right. The skin complaints are viewed not as an illness in their own right — not in fact as an illness of the skin — but as a disturbance of the whole constitution, which is expressed through the skin.

Whether the diagnosis is "eczema" or "psoriasis," the homeopath will always look for a possible cause or rather for the trigger. To choose the correct remedy, it's clearly important to note how the complaints are expressed, such as how the skin rash looks, whether it itches, burns, or hurts. The circumstances in which the complaints worsen or improve are also important. But most of all, it's the person behind the complaints that interests us. Who is this child and what's the matter with him or her?

Many skin complaints can be treated successfully with homeopathy, although often a lot of patience is required — especially when the complaints are long-standing, and they occur frequently in the family. But homeopathic treatment — together with conventional medical care if necessary — takes hold at the roots, so that we achieve not just a pretty appearance but also an improved sense of general well-being. The following example illustrates this.

Warts

Never before had I seen so many warts together! Suzan certainly had more than 200 all over her tiny body. The family doctor had said that he could remove them. To cut out a single wart is painful enough, but 200 — and in a three-year-old girl!

"Did something special happen before the warts appeared?" I asked. Suzan had no complaints from the warts and was otherwise as fit as a fiddle. Yet I needed to find a way into the case so I could choose the right remedy from around 100 remedies that can cure warts. "The only thing is that she's had a very sad time," answered her mother. "Her father, who she's very close to, had to go away on business for several weeks. She had great difficulty coming to terms with this. She put a brave face on it, but I noticed how much she missed him."

243

I looked up the case in my repertory, the book in which all symptoms are listed together with the corresponding homeopathic remedies. To my surprise, it listed *Natrium carbonicum*, which is the principal remedy for grief at the father's absence. The quiet, sensitive character of Suzan fitted this very well. She liked the taste of the globuli that I immediately put on her tongue. Children often feel very clearly what's good for them.

Six weeks later, Suzan proudly and cheerfully showed me her arms, legs, and abdomen. There were still a few small bumps to be seen, but most of the warts had disappeared. What pleased me even more was her mother's comment that Suzan was back to her old self, cheerful and open. As if the disappearance of the warts had lifted a weight off her shoulders.

Index

This index lists important characteristics with their corresponding remedies. This doesn't mean that children always have these characteristics, but that the characteristics are often found in the remedy pictures listed. Obviously, these characteristics can also occur in other child types.

Absent-minded /
scatter-brained: *Agaricus, Alumina, Barium carbonicum, Helium, Hydrogenium, Medorrhinum, Opium, Thuja*

Aggressive: *Ammonium carbonicum, Anacardium, Belladonna, Chamomilla, Lachesis, Lycopodium, Mercurius, Nux vomica*

Attention-seeking: *Calcarea sulfurica, Hyoscyamus, Lachesis, Lithium phosphoricum, Saccharum*

Collect, tendency to: *Arsenicum album, Sulfur*

Compulsive: *Arsenicum album, Beryllium, Carcinosinum, Cuprum, Thuja*

Concentration, poor: *Agaricus, Alumina, Barium carbonicum, Helium, Hydrogenium, Lithium metallicum, Lithium phosphoricum, Opium, Saccharum, Thuja, Tuberculinum*

Conformist: *Beryllium, Calcarea carbonica, Carcinosinum, Lac caninum, Magnesium muriaticum, Magnesium phosphoricum, Manganum, Pulsatilla, Silicea*

Confused: *Agaricus, Alumina, Borax, Opium*

Contrary: *Anacardium, Antimonium crudum, Belladonna, Chamomilla, Cina, Lycopodium, Mercurius, Nux vomica*

Demanding: *Agaricus, Apis mellifica, Belladonna, Chamomilla, Cina, Lithium metallicum, Lithium* *phosphoricum, Mercurius, Saccharum, Stramonium, Tuberculinum*

Disheveled (careless about appearance): *Sulfur*

Dominant: *Arnica, Aurum, Cuprum, Ferrum, Lachesis, Lycopodium, Mercurius, Nux vomica*

Eager to learn: *Aurum, Carcinosinum, Lachesis, Phosphorus, Silicea*

Fear of being abandoned: *Magnesium carbonicum, Magnesium muriaticum, Magnesium phosphoricum*

Fearful: *Arsenicum album, Barium carbonicum, Calcarea carbonica, Calcarea phosphorica, Calcarea silicata, Calcarea sulfurica, Lac caninum, Lithium metallicum, Lithium phosphoricum, Opium, Stramonium*

Forward: *Aconitum, Anacardium, Antimonium crudum, Arnica, Aurum, Belladonna, Chamomilla, Cina, Cuprum, Ferrum, Lachesis, Lycopodium, Mercurius, Nux vomica, Sulfur*

Helpful: *Aconitum, Arnica, Aurum, Beryllium, Calcarea phosphorica, Carcinosinum, Causticum, Lithium phosphoricum, Manganum, Natrium carbonicum, Natrium muriaticum, Nux vomica, Phosphorus, Pulsatilla*

Irritable, quickly: (see "Aggressive")

Jealous: *Calcarea sulfurica, Hyoscyamus, Lachesis, Lycopodium, Saccharum*

Leadership qualities: (see "Dominant")

Mean: *Anacardium, Chamomilla, Cina, Lachesis, Lycopodium, Medorrhinum, Mercurius*

Nasty: (see "Mean")

Index

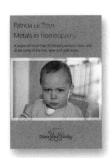

Patricia Le Roux
Metals in Homeopathy

A review of more than 50 clinical paediatric cases from the iron, silver- and gold series

384 pages, hb, € 38.-

"Patricia Le Roux has again written an excellent book on homeopathy and pediatrics. She is a very good clinician with the ability to express her experiences and ideas in a very clear fashion. ... You will be convinced that this book is well worth buying." Jan Scholten

Metals have long been used in homeopathy and there exists a rich library of classical literature detailing the properties and uses of a range of well-known metal polychrests. Building on our established knowledge base and on the insights of Scholten and Sankaran, this book offers a wealth of information about a very wide range of metal remedies and their neighbors from the iron, silver and gold series of the periodic table.

Patricia Le Roux provides over fifty inspiring cases from her pediatric practice to illustrate her understanding of the key themes and the clinical use of these fifty-four important elements. Through these case examples, she demonstrates the extraordinary role that metals and their allies can play in helping children realize their full potential – to succeed in whatever projects, careers or lifestyles they undertake, to become genuine artists.

The book provides an invaluable reference source both for practitioners treating children and for those keen to deepen and broaden their understanding of these key remedies from the mineral kingdom. It also offers compelling evidence for the usefulness of homeopathic treatment within the realm of Integrative Medicine.

"Patricia is very good at looking for and finding the essence, in her patients and in the remedies. She has a great talent for incorporating the new theories in homeopathy and elaborating on them. And she has a great talent for successfully applying those theories to her patients and ... to write down her experiences in a precise and clear way."

Jan Scholten

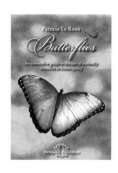

Patricia Le Roux
Butterflies

An innovative guide to the use of butterfly remedies in homeopathy

144 pages, hb, € 18.-

The well-known French paediatrician Patricia Le Roux ventures in this book into the virtually unknown territory of butterfly remedies in homeopathy. She has found these remedies particularly useful among hyperactive (ADHD) children who are lively, agitated, restless and mercurial. In these "butterfly children", there is often a strong feeling of being abandoned, especially by their father or mother, which is experienced as loss of imposed authority and safe boundaries.

Butterfly remedies also have a common theme of metamorphosis – the desire to dress up. They enjoy masks and are confused about their own identity. The author has found these remedies very effective too in various skin problems, such as urticaria or eczema.

The book contains provings, cases and concise essences of 13 butterfly and moth remedies: The California Sister, The Tailed Jay, The Lilac Beauty, The Processional Caterpillar, The Brown Tail Moth, The Brimstone, The Death's Head Hawkmoth, The Blue Morpho, The European Peacock, The Marsh Fritillary, The Cabbage White, The Small Tortoiseshell and The Fox Moth. These different remedies are clearly differentiated and vividly described, paving the way for exciting new prescription possibilities.

"A wonderful small book by one of our best homeopathic explorers. I learned a lot – and now see people who need butterflies everywhere! Highly recommended."
David Kent Warkentin

"Patricia Le Roux has again produced a very fine book. The pictures of the butterflies are very lively and portray the essence."
Jan Scholten

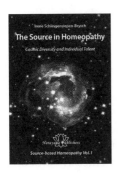

Irene Schlingensiepen-Brysch
The Source in Homeopathy

Cosmic Diversity and Individual Talent

Source-based Homeopathy Vol. I

144 pages, hb, € 18.-

The knowledge of the most effective remedy is to be found in the subconscious of every human being. The adept homeopath can facilitate the individual's access to this hidden knowledge.

Dr. Schlingensiepen has laid the foundation for this innovative approach through years of carefully documented case-taking and systematic investigation of the follow-ups.

Using 24 remedy pictures of cosmic origin – such as Sol, Helium, Positronium, Meteorite, Brass, Volcano, precious stones, and Geyser – she shows how we can accompany our patients on the journey into their unconscious and help them to name the source of their remedy. This may even be a remedy that is so far unknown to homeopathy, yet which is nevertheless capable of bringing about profound healing, even in serious illness.

"Irene Schlingensiepen-Brysch is a scientist who has managed to retain her scientific approach as a homeopath, in order to search out the unwritten laws of a successful prescription. In Irene the right hemisphere is connected to the left, analysis encounters synthesis, east meets west."

Harry van der Zee

"Irene Schlingensiepen-Brysch carefully, unwaveringly, and persistently follows the stream of words and gestures coming from her patients, upstream to the healing source. The way is radically new ... A source of inspiration and an example of homeopathy practised with integrity and to a high scientific standard."

Uta Santos-König

"I recommend this book to all homeopaths. It can trigger a very deep understanding of the effectiveness of remedies, their essences, and sources."

Jan Scholten

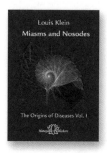

Louis Klein
Miasms and Nosodes

The Origins of Diseases - Volume I

528 pages, hb, € 49.-

Louis Klein is one of the leading homeopaths world-wide. His latest book on miasms and nosodes is a ground-breaking pioneer work in the field of homeopathy.

On the basis of his broad clinical experience, Louis Klein attributes many known remedies to miasmatic states. A miasmatic state becomes the core idea around which similar remedies are grouped. For example the Tetanus miasm comprises not only Tetanus nosode but also remedies like Hypericum, An-gustura, Helodrilus, Tellurium. It is clinically linked also with tetanic syndromes, spasms or even convulsions. This new classification of miasmatic remedies is highly practical and opens a new chapter in homeopathy, demystifying and redefining the existing miasms, while adding several important new ones. It also introduces new remedies like Johneinum and Helodrilus, which he has proved extensively. So Louis Klein's work on miasms and nosodes is indeed a homeopathic milestone.

In this first volume Louis Klein presents in-depth information on Burkholderiales including the Pertussis miasm; Clostridiales including the Tetanus miasm; Corynebacteria including the Diphtheria miasm; Mycobacteria including the Tubercular and Leprosy miasms, plus the newly proven remedy Johneinum, linked to the Crohn's disease miasm; Enterobacteriales including the Bach Bowel Nosodes, the Typhoid and Yersinia miasms; and Parasitic Protozoa and Parasitic miasms including the Malaria and Toxoplasmosis miasms.

All this practical information is illustrated throughout with excellent case examples from two decades of homeopathic practice, which speak for themselves. This book is in a class of its own. As Rajan Sankaran is known for plant remedies and Jan Scholten for the periodic table, Louis Klein will be known for miasms and nosodes.

"Nosodes have the aspect of being vague, not precisely defined. Lou Klein has the capacity to work with this vagueness very effectively. He knows how to extract the essence of the remedy from provings, from natural history and especially from patients. He is able to make the vague more exact. This book is the first to do this successfully in homeopathy. I see this book as a must for every homeopath."
Jan Scholten

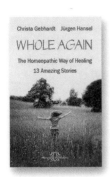

Gebhardt / Hansel
Whole Again

The Homeopathic Way of Healing

13 Amazing Stories

224 pages, pb, € 18.-

An enchanting introduction to homeopathy as it has never been made before. 13 selected cases from world-renowned homeopathic physicians such as Rajan Sankaran and Jan Scholten were independently verified. The authors were so dedicated to this task that they travelled around the world in order not to have to rely solely on the therapists' accounts. They visited all of the cured patients in their homes and let them speak in their own surroundings. This lends an authenticity that has hitherto not existed in homeopathic literature.

The authors: A sensitive homeopathic physician and his wife, a journalist, with astonishing skill. They took it upon themselves to record especially interesting, exciting or touching life stories of patients who all share something in common: They were healed by homeopathy and experienced what this wonderful approach to medicine can bring about - to become "whole again".

What may appear to be simply a stroke of luck in an individual case does indeed prove itself as a method that can be learned. It can thus be understood by the reader how each therapist found the necessary remedy. We become acquainted with people such as the Indian executive, who was partially paralyzed by a herniated disc and was soon able to walk again after a dose of his remedy; or Maria, who was born with a handicap but able to perform well in school with the help of homeopathy; or a woman from the Netherlands, whose remedy helped her to feel her body again after 30 years of numbness resulting from a severe burning incident.

The book depicts the entire scope of modern homeopathy and is thus of great current interest. The experienced therapist will also become acquainted with new remedy pictures. A highly interesting work which is sure to win new friends of homeopathy and which we hope will find a wide following!

"One of the most beautiful - maybe the most beautiful book about homeopathy."
Journal „Natur und Medizin"

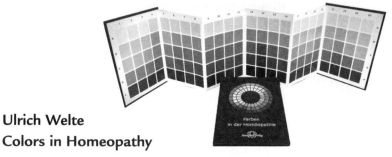

Ulrich Welte
Colors in Homeopathy

Color charts and textbook with repertory, € 48.-

The color preference expresses the inner state of a patient directly, and as such it is a significant and specific homeopathic symptom. It has been helpful to indicate or confirm the correct diagnosis of a remedy in many cases. 18 years of clinical experience in thousands of cases stand behind this publication.

The color preference as a homeopathic symptom was discovered by H.V. Müller in 1985. The 120 colors presented in this book were selected according to clinical relevance and allow us to assess the color preference with sufficient accuracy. The corresponding remedies can be looked up in the color/remedy list like in a repertory. The printed version comprises more than 1000 well-confirmed remedies. The list of the website is updated regularly with the latest clinical findings.

"The color preference is a significant and effective symptom. It's effective in the sense that it can give the indication or confirmation of a diagnosis in many cases. The color preference is a peculiar symptom expressing the inner state of the patient, which is the state of the remedy. And it's a very specific symptom. The table designed by Ulrich Welte is the best usable I've seen till now. All colors are clear and accurately standardized, so it can be used in the future without ambiguity."

Jan Scholten

"I am fully convinced that Dr Mueller should be made a homeopathic saint! I can hardly imagine the good karma that should be bestowed on him from the results of this wonderful work. Through it I have travelled down unexpected paths to the similimum and have procured cures I could never have hoped for with the regular homeopathic method. The wonder of color selection has led me to choose medicines I would never have previously used with great success as well as confirming effective medicines where before I would have been riddled with doubt."

Peter Tumminello

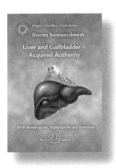

Rosina Sonnenschmidt
Liver and Gallbladder - Acquired Authority

128 pages, hb, € 29.-

The place where disease manifests within the organ system is deeply significant. This is the site of conflict, but where there is conflict there is also the opportunity for resolution - and in resolution lies cure.

The liver is the focus of the second volume in the series Organ - Conflict - Cure by Rosina Sonnenschmidt. The author shows us the energetic significance of the liver discussing its symbolism, the liver temperament and spiritual matters whilst outlining the place of the liver in the historical context of alchemy and its importance in Traditional Chinese Medicine.

The issues associated with the liver are 'acquired authority' - the personal power that one develops in the course of one's life - creativity, humour and drive. If the energy of the liver is suppressed, for example by low self-esteem, the result can be aggression and a wide variety of physical conditions ranging from rheumatism and diabetes to cirrhosis of the liver.

As well as providing detailed information about the structure, function and pathology of the liver, the author gives much invaluable practical advice on treating liver and gallbladder complaints based on her many years as a holistic therapist.

Areas covered include:
- nutrition
- deacidification and detoxification
- herbal remedies
- cleansing the liver and gallbladder
- homeopathy
- extensive section on homeopathic therapeutic remedies

Many schools of thought are drawn on throughout the book, the emphasis being on the miasmatic point of view.

This is a comprehensive and fascinating book that deals with every aspect of the liver in an easily accessible style.

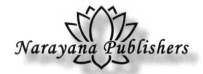

Blumenplatz 2, 79400 Kandern, Germany
Tel: +49 7626-9749700, Fax: +49 7626-9749709
info@narayana-publishers.eu

At our online shop
www.narayana-publishers.eu
you will find all English and German homeopathic titles
as well as information on seminars with leading homeopaths.
We offer informative reading samples for each title.
We deliver books to homeopathic schools and training
courses at special rates.

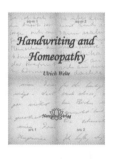

Ulrich Welte

Handwriting and Homeopathy

344 pages, hb, no. 00671, € 28.-

Personality structure expresses itself in handwriting. Handwriting is a frozen image of motion patterns. So handwriting is a significant clinical background symptom of great depth. It is well worth learning to read this 'script inside the script'. 20 years of clinical experience and in thousands of cases, handwriting has shown its homeopathic efficiency as a confirmatory symptom, or it pointed directly to the correct diagnosis of a remedy.

This book is a reference work to compare handwritings in homeopathic practice. It contains 750 handwriting samples of 315 remedies. Numerous case descriptions illustrate the usefulness of this new symptom and serve as a practical guide to its successful application. The cases show how often the symptoms of handwriting and color preference helped in finding a good remedy. One will also notice how often the series and stages of Jan Scholten's interpretation of the periodic table proved true. Rajan Sankaran's recent and earlier findings were frequently verified. So our advice would be to study these ideas thoroughly. They are highly rewarding, and it will also make the case descriptions more understandable.